THE NATURE OF NURSING

A Definition and Its Implications
for Practice, Research,
and Education

REFLECTIONS AFTER 25 YEARS

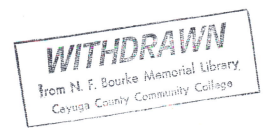

THE NATURE OF NURSING

A Definition and Its Implications for Practice, Research, and Education

REFLECTIONS AFTER 25 YEARS

Virginia A. Henderson, AM, RN

National League for Nursing Press • New York

Pub. No. 15-2346

Copyright © 1991
National League for Nursing
350 Hudson Street, New York, NY 10014

ISBN 0-88737-494-8

This book was set in Garamond by Publications Development Company. The editor was
Sally J. Barhydt; the designer was Allan Graubard. Northeastern Press was the printer
and binder.

The cover was designed by Lillian Welsh.

This book contains the unabridged reprint of *The Nature of Nursing*, published by the
Macmillan Company in 1966.

Printed in the United States of America.

Contents

Preface

*L*ike the first edition of this book, the new edition reflects the personal viewpoint of the author. After reviewing the first edition for publication by the National League for Nursing Press in 1991, I concluded that, in the main, after twenty-five years it still reflects my concept of "the nature of nursing." If I were writing a comparable statement today, I would make some changes or emphasize certain points that were not emphasized in the 1966 edition. But rather than rewrite the whole book, I decided to comment in what I have chosen to call an "addendum" to each chapter. These addenda enable me to give the changes in my views and to explain my opinions or why I question them.

It has been my good fortune to meet, to know, to work with experts in many aspects of health service. I am indebted to them for what they have taught me.

Readers who are interested can get some idea of the nature and range of my sources of information if they use the extensive text *Principles and Practice of Nursing* (6th ed., Macmillan Co., 1978) written with eighteen joint authors and expert nurses.

Virginia Henderson
New Haven, Connecticut
1991

Preface to the First Edition

*T*his small volume is the expression of a viewpoint on nursing with an attempt to identify the persons and experiences that most influenced it. The contents grew out of a Clare Dennison Memorial Lecture at the University of Rochester School of Nursing in the spring of 1964. A condensed version was published in the *American Journal of Nursing* in August 1964. Because study of the writings of others is one kind of experience that has affected the development of certain opinions expressed here, many books and articles are cited. Only by reference to them can the reader of this text fully understand some ideas that could be presented in essence only.

Since this is in the nature of a professional memoir, or testament, it is written in the first person. In trying to show how I have come to regard the nursing function, and how this concept has affected my idea of nursing practice, research, and education, I decided that the first person was the most appropriate form to use.

Much of what I have to say about nursing practice has been presented in more detail in my last revision of Miss Bertha Harmer's text, *The Principles and Practice of Nursing,* and in the ICN's booklet, *Basic Principles of Nursing Care.* Certain comments on nursing research are more elaborately treated in

Nursing Research—A Survey and Assessment, by Leo W. Simmons and me, and in our related publications. The implications for nursing education in my definition of the nurse's function have not been presented elsewhere, so they are given more emphasis than those for practice or research.

Because nurses are predominantly women, I refer to the nurse as "she," and by the same token I refer to the physician as "he," but this usage does not mean that I would not welcome a more equal distribution of the sexes in all the major health fields.

Interest expressed by readers of the *Journal* article leads me to hope that this expanded version may be of some value in the nurse's continuing effort to serve mankind more effectively and to enjoy a greater satisfaction in her work.

V. H.
1966

Foreword

Virginia Henderson was breakfasting with several ardent admirers at a home care convention a couple years ago, when we queried her for the umptieth time about getting *The Nature of Nursing* back into print. Her retort was quintessential Virginia: "I do wish people would stop talking about that book as though my concept of nursing stopped developing over 20 years ago."

I lingered after breakfast to ask if she would be willing to update *Nature* for re-publication, with assistance. Virginia said she would. Excited by the prospect of seeing a new edition of the book, I walked out into the lobby and ran smack into Pam Maraldo. Pam shared my excitement and immediately agreed that the National League for Nursing Press would take on the project.

Virginia Henderson was true to her word in updating the manuscript, though she accepted very little help. The League worked diligently with Virginia to bring the revised edition to publication. We owe both a great deal for reviving this classic for a new generation of nurses.

Only Virginia, who speaks of nursing as "of the head and of the hands and of the heart," could capture our profession with such elegant simplicity. Her essence of caring and egalitarian philosophy soar from the pages. This great lady of nursing teaches us by her example to accept and embrace change throughout our lives. The book follows: let her speak for herself.

Margaret J. Cushman
President, VNA Group, Inc.
Visiting Nurse And Home Care, Inc.
Plainville, Connecticut

1

The Search for an Official Definition of Nursing

*I*t is self-evident that an occupation, and especially a profession, whose services affect human life must define its function.

Inevitably we go back to Florence Nightingale, whose most often quoted work, *Notes on Nursing — What It Is and What It Is Not,*[1] was published in 1859. She said, in essence, that what nursing has to do is to ". . . put the patient in the best condition for nature to act upon him." There is no doubt that Miss Nightingale's concept influenced the development of modern nursing more than any other. Some nurses still cite this definition as the one they find most helpful.

But, with the passage of the Nurse Registration Act in England and state nurse practice acts in the United States around the turn of the century, it was necessary to describe nursing in such a way as to protect the public and the nurse. This was a period of rapid advance in medical technology and expansion of hospital nursing programs. However, there was not an equivalent advance in nursing competence. As late as 1930 students were regularly staffing hospital nursing services, the seniors often acting as head nurses in charge of clinical units or wards.* Graduates were to be found in visiting nurse agencies; a few worked in schools and physicians' offices, but most were private practitioners in homes and hospitals. None of these situations was conducive to the development of clinical expertness, although many nurses acquired a fine self-taught art of nursing. For these and other reasons, most legal definitions of the period implied that the nurse operated under the supervision of a physician. They failed to identify the aspect of her work that was independent or self-directed.

Understandably the idea of the nurse as being merely the physician's assistant has never been satisfying to the occupation as a whole, nor is it in line with nurses' insistence that they direct nursing schools and services. Many articles could be cited to this effect, although in surveying the literature I found no concerted objection to the prevailing tone of the nurse practice acts until recent years.

In 1933 and 1934 Effie J. Taylor raised the same question I am now discussing—what is the nature of nursing?[2,3] She accepted the definition of nursing as "adapting prescribed therapy and preventive treatment to the specific physical and psychic needs of the individual." But she also said, "The real depths of nursing can only be made known through ideals, love, sympathy, knowledge, and culture, expressed through the practice of artistic procedures and relationships." In these statements Miss Taylor anticipated some of the current emphases on patient-centered, individualized care and on the importance of a liberal education for the nurse.

I suppose there were rumblings throughout the first half of this century, but after World War II there seems to have been an explosion of discontent with the ambiguous position of nursing.

In 1946 the American Nurses' Association asked certain nursing leaders to formulate definitions. One response to this

---

* Few realize that the graduate staff nurse in hospitals was an innovation of the twenties following World War I. (See Best, Ella: *The Use of the Graduate Nurse on a Staff Basis.* New York, American Nurses' Association, 1931, lv 22.)

was a small leaflet that Annie W. Goodrich published and distributed at her own expense.[4] Slightly modified, it appeared later in the *American Journal of Nursing*.[5]

About this time Esther Lucile Brown was commissioned by the National Nursing Council to study the needs of society for nursing. Her report in 1948 is entitled *Nursing for the Future*.[6] In this volume she cites a definition formulated by nurse experts who were asked by the National League of Nursing Education to meet for this purpose. The resulting statement of the nurse's function is excellent but so general that any health worker might claim that it is also his function. In connection with Miss Brown's survey three regional conferences were held; a mimeographed report of them is entitled *A Thousand Think Together*.[7] At the Washington conference a small committee, of which I was a member, presented a more specific definition that was, in fact, my point of view modified by the thinking of others in the group. As far as I know the statement was never used, except indirectly.

In 1950 the American Nurses' Association embarked on a five-year investigation of the nurse's function. Nearly half a million dollars was raised by nurses to conduct studies in 17 states. Each was reported separately, but they were summarized by Everett and Helen MacGill Hughes and Irwin Deutscher under the title *Twenty Thousand Nurses Tell Their Story*.[8]

Whether or not these investigations give us a satisfying description of the nurse function is open to question. However, there can be no doubt that those who have read the inclusive report know far more than they did before about what nurses were actually doing in the fifties, how they regarded themselves and their work, how their associates regarded them, and how the public looked upon nurses and nursing.

In 1955 the Board of Directors of the American Nurses' Association approved the definition of nursing practice submitted by its Committee on Legislation. This remains the official statement as published again in 1962.[9] It is designed for inclusion in nurse practice acts and reads as follows:

Practice of Nursing

    1. The practice of professional nursing means the performance for compensation of any act in the observation, care, and counsel of the ill, injured, or infirm, or in the maintenance of health or prevention of illness of others, or in the supervision and teaching of other personnel, or the administration of medications and treatment as prescribed by a licensed physician or dentist; requiring substantial specialized judgment and skill and based on knowledge and application of the principles of biological, physical, and social science. The foregoing shall not be deemed to include acts of diagnosis or prescription of therapeutic or corrective measures.

    2. The practice of practical nursing means the performance for compensation of selected acts in the care of the ill, injured, or infirm under the direction of a registered professional nurse or a licensed physician or a licensed dentist; and not requiring the substantial specialized skill, judgment, and knowledge required in professional nursing.[10]

I think this statement, although still very general and all inclusive, suggests at least that the nurse can observe, care for, and counsel the patient and can supervise other health personnel without herself being supervised by the physician. She can give only such medications and treatments as are prescribed by a physician and must refrain from diagnosing, prescribing, and correcting. This 1955 statement does certainly imply a more independent function than did that formulated in 1932 and published again as "Professional Nursing Defined" in 1937, but it is still unspecific.[11] Nathan Hershey, assistant director of the Health Law Center, University of Pittsburgh, in one of a series of articles on "The Law and the Nurse" published in 1962, said that nurse practice acts describe practice "in a general way."[12] Milton J. Lesnik, an authority on nurse jurisprudence, has called attention to the same weakness in these acts.[13, 14] *

---

    * In 1948 Pearl Castile, a nurse educator, analyzed the effect of these acts on schools of nursing. She concluded that state laws had not been revised as nursing education was upgraded and that they were not serving the purpose for which they

While the official statements on nursing may serve the purpose for which they are intended, there is abundant evidence that over the years they have not satisfied everyone. Physicians interested in nursing, such as Dr. Osler, have tried to say what they expected or hoped for from the nurse. Dr. Osler urged us to nurse the man as well as the patient and suggested that the nurse is, to some extent, a mother substitute; certain present-day psychiatrists have also cast us in this role. Another physician, Dr. J. C. Meakins, showed dissatisfaction with current statements when he said in 1948, "Nursing must be defined."[15] He thought it should be described in such a way that the duties of nurses at all levels would be defined and the nurse could be protected from having to assume legal responsibility for non-nursing procedures. He advised nurses to control their own destinies and said that nurses of that decade needed a little of the "divine madness" that motivated early leaders.

In recent years, with the development of recognized, certified or registered grades of nursing personnel, the difficulty of defining function is compounded. This may account, more than any other circumstance, for the fact that in a national survey recently reported more persons recommended research on the nurse's function, role, and status than on any other question.[16] During the fifties, thousands of nurses participated in the development of statements on functions, standards, and qualifications for practice in the various fields of nursing represented by the following sections of the American Nurses' Association: Counselors, Executive Secretaries, and Registrars Section; Educational Administrators, Consultants, and Teachers Section; Nursing Service Administrators Section; Office Nurses Section; Occupational Health Nursing Section; Private Duty Nurses Section; and Public Health Nurses Section. These are valuable documents and can be found in the *American Journal of Nursing*

---

were designed. She maintained that not one act was sufficiently strong to eliminate the weak school characterized in Esther Lucile Brown's report as "socially undesirable." Castile, Pearl: *Nurse Practice Acts, Their Effect upon Schools of Nursing* (Ed. Dissertation). Stanford University, Palo Alto, Calif., 1948.

during the last decade. From them might be distilled a highly significant definition of nursing, but in their present form they offer only a diffuse list of widely differing functions.

To summarize, major efforts have been made by individuals, small groups, and organized nursing to formulate a statement of its function, but we must conclude that this is still unfinished business. Perhaps it is one of these perennial problems that will always exist because conditions change from one era to the next and change with the culture, or the nature, of a society. However, as long as official definitions are unsatisfying to nurses, or too general to protect the nurse and the public or to guide practice, research, and education, individual nurses will continue to seek statements that fulfill their needs. As children are now taught to say, I would like to "share" with you *my* search and my conclusions.

ADDENDUM
THE SEARCH FOR AN OFFICIAL
DEFINITION OF NURSING

In spite of the fact that generations of nurses have tried to define it, "the nature of nursing" remains a question. Florence Nightingale in the last century dramatically reduced the death rate in the military hospitals during the Crimean War with nursing as she understood it, but I doubt whether her definition was generally known then or now.

Florence Nightingale thought that nurses "put patients in the best state" for *nature* to cure them. She said that neither doctors nor nurses cured people. Nothing has been more discussed in nursing circles this century and in this country than the function of the nurse, and nursing research since 1950 has been focused on this question.

If I were writing today about an official definition of nursing, I would put even more stress on it than I did in 1966. It seems to me we are no nearer a consensus now than we were then. One difference today, however, is that many nursing schools offer courses on "the theory of nursing" and on "the nursing process," and this topic has become the context for seeking a definition.

Asked to write an article on nursing process, I reviewed the extensive literature on the subject. I concluded that it was differentiated from the *medical* process by the language employed rather than by the steps making up the "process." Although I think that far too much time and energy has been devoted to nursing process and the theory of nursing, were I writing *The Nature of Nursing* today I would feel obliged to include a discussion of both. I would urge nurses to read what others write on the subjects, hoping that it would help them clarify their own thoughts.

Having visited numerous countries in recent years, noting the great disparity between the numbers and preparation of the nursing personnel, I find it more and more difficult to promote acceptance of a universal definition of nursing. Perhaps we should accept the conclusion that it depends on the resources of the country involved and the needs of the people it serves.

In countries such as England and Holland where nurse mid-wives deliver the majority of infants, the concept of these health care providers differs from the concept of midwives in the United States where nurse midwives deliver a small proportion of infants. This disparity helps explain the difference in the relationship of doctors and nurse midwives in these countries and ultimately in the definition of their roles.

2

Development of a Personal Concept

*M*y interpretation of the nurse's function is the synthesis of many influences—some positive, some negative. In chronological order I will identify those experiences I think most significant. First I would like to emphasize that I am not presenting my point of view as one with which I expect you to agree. Rather I would urge every nurse to develop her own concept, otherwise she is merely imitating others or acting under authority. In my own case I felt as though I were steering an uncharted course until I resolved certain doubts about my true function.

Most of my basic training was in a general hospital where, for the nurse, technical competence, speed of performance, and a "professional" (actually an impersonal) manner were stressed. We were introduced to nursing as a series of almost unrelated procedures, beginning with an unoccupied bed and progressing to aspiration of body cavities, for instance. Ability to catheterize a patient in this era seemed to qualify a student for so-called night duty where, without any previous experience in the administration of a service, she might have the entire care of as many as thirty sick souls and bodies.

An authoritarian type of medicine was practiced in this hospital. Physicians who lectured to student nurses simply compressed and simplified the didactic instruction they gave medical students. They usually presented watertight diagnoses with textbook programs of therapy and cut-and-dried prognoses. In those days not even lip-service was given "patient-centered care," "family health service," "comprehensive care," or "rehabilitation."

But there was, for me, an influence in those early student days that tended to negate this mechanistic approach. Annie W. Goodrich was Dean of my school, the Army School of Nursing. Whenever she visited our unit, she lifted our sights above techniques and routines. With her broad experience in hospitals, in public health agencies, and educational institutions, she saw nursing as a "world-wide social activity," a creative and constructive force in society. Having a powerful intellect and boundless compassion for humanity, she never failed to infect us with "the ethical significance of nursing." This is the title she later chose for her collected papers, and it could not have been more apt for it was the essence of her teaching.[17]

Miss Goodrich often expressed full awareness of the physician's immeasurable contribution to social welfare and had a surprising knowledge of current therapies. Nevertheless, I attribute to her my early discontent with the regimentalized patient care in which I participated and the concept of nursing as merely ancillary to medicine. Although Miss Goodrich always presented us with the highest aim for nursing, she left us to translate it into concrete acts, and I needed someone to "show me"—as Liza Doolittle sang, when words had ceased to be enough for her. Dr. Osler's greatest contribution may well have been his insistence that medical students have the opportunity to see their teachers *practice* medicine. I seldom, if ever, saw graduate nurses *practice* nursing—never my teachers. Their teaching was in a classroom.

While it is true that as a student I was clinically self-taught for the most part, in the army hospital I had the privilege of

nursing sick and wounded soldiers who were notably coura-
geous and appreciative. I learned to serve in an atmosphere
where the nurse, as a representative of society, felt indebted to
the patient. The soldier patient demanded little, but the nurse
felt that the most she could do was not enough, and therefore
the nurse-patient relationship was a warm and generous one.
The atmosphere in certain affiliated civil hospitals offered a
distinct contrast, and so, in this respect, we thought our student
nursing experience special, if not unique.

Professional and nonprofessional literature in recent de-
cades abounds in criticism of hospitals. Their present burden is
so great that it seems ungenerous to point to such publications.
Some criticize the nursing care; others question many services
hospitals offer. Elizabeth Barnes, in a small volume, *People in
Hospital,* summarizes the findings of eighteen groups studying
hospitals in Canada, Finland, France, Germany, Italy, Spain,
Switzerland, the United Kingdom, and the United States.[18] Although this descriptive and judicial document shows up many
weaknesses, it also notes that "hospitals contain and cope with
the disorder and distress of illness which the community itself
cannot tolerate."

Present-day hospitals as represented in this survey seem to
offer a wide range of service by type and quality. For example,
some permit families to move in with patients and help care for
them, while others prohibit even parents visiting their children.
One hospital is reported to have weekly interprofessional ward
conferences attended by all members of the clinical team with,
preferably, the head nurse presiding; but the statement follows
that "meetings of this kind would be incompatible with the
social structure of some hospitals." Certain hospitals represented have open days that encourage public interest and observation; others discourage public involvement.

Jan de Hartog has shown that in this decade conditions in a
hospital of one of the wealthiest regions of the United States
can rival in horror those found in the Dark Ages.[19] He does not,
however, attribute the state of the hospital to the inhumanity of

medical personnel primarily but rather to the apathy of the public and to the governing board that failed to provide conditions under which such personnel could operate effectively. He is as compassionate toward doctors and nurses as he is toward patients, for he sees all of them as victims of prejudice and a totally inadequate system.

No doubt many persons fear hospitalization, and others, unless they are desperately ill, feel apologetic about asking overburdened doctors and nurses to care for them. Social scientists are vocal on this score. Esther Lucile Brown in a series of books with the over-all title *Newer Dimensions of Patient Care* is an ardent and effective spokesman for the public.[20, 21, 22] These publications suggest changes in the general hospital that have been effected in certain psychiatric hospitals in which the goal is the establishment of a therapeutic environment.[23, 24]

Medical and nursing faculties, realizing the limitations of institutional care, sporadically in the past and more generally at present, have offered their students (and some staff members) experience outside the hospital.[25, 26, 27, 28] Programs that attempt to meet the total needs of patients as they move from inpatient to outpatient services demonstrate some of the gaps in hospital care as it exists today. The findings of Dr. George Reader, Doris Schwartz, and their associates at the New York-Cornell Medical Center seem to indicate that the ambulatory patients treated in the outpatient department are, to be quite specific, unable to use correctly at home the very drugs prescribed for them by the physician.[29, 30] Other studies point to the relative inadequacy of written directions as a means of helping patients carry out prescribed therapy.

The president of a large university, speaking to me of medical education there, said that he and the medical and nursing faculties sometimes wondered whether medical personnel with a patient-centered approach could be produced within the hospital setting because so many of its practices are contrary to the best interests of patients. Esther Lucile Brown in *Newer Dimensions of Patient Care* suggests some radical changes that must be made in the hospital if it is to be patient-centered. Dr. Crew quotes Miss Nightingale as saying, "Hospitals are only an intermediate stage of civilization. . . ."[31] But this has been a digression on the limitations of our major institutions for medical care, and I should return to my student experiences.

Part of my preparation for nursing was in a psychiatric affiliation that might have supplied me with many of the human relation skills I needed—those, in fact, all health workers need. There, hopefully, I might have seen an individualized program for patients that I failed to see in the general hospital. Actually, I learned names for supposed disease entities and treatments for them, most of which have been, or should have been, discarded. The chief value of this affiliation was that it gave me some appreciation of the extent and nature of mental illness. I acquired little or no understanding of the role a nurse might play in preventing or curing it. The following is an example of how completely I failed to grasp my function as a psychiatric nurse.

I was assigned the care of a large and very sick woman from a socially prominent family. We were alone in a short wing of the hospital. She was extremely negative and assaultive. She had attacked several nurses and had injured one by pinning her behind a door. I was frightened during this assignment until I found that by playing the part of a "handmaiden," speaking archaic English, and addressing my patient as "Your Majesty," I could get her to do anything. No one came to her aid—or mine—and so I left her even more deeply entrenched in the world of fantasy than she was when she fell into my ignorant hands. Only years later did I realize how untherapeutic my approach had been.

While my psychiatric nursing experience left me with a sense of failure, a pediatric affiliation with the Boston Floating Hospital had the opposite effect, for there I was introduced to patient-centered care, although this term was not used then. In that hospital we were regularly assigned patients, not tasks. Each of us cared for three sick infants or children. When the student with whom we were paired was "off duty," we would care for her three patients as well as our own. Under such circumstances we acquired considerable understanding of our charges and their needs, and we were greatly attached to them. The director of nurses and the able head nurses, who in this hospital were graduates, encouraged a warm relationship between patients and students.* Here we saw "tender loving care" before the label was invented. Unfortunately we did not see demonstrated the importance of bringing the mothers or fathers into the hospital with the sick child. While we glimpsed patient-centered care, it was not family-centered. We knew little or nothing of the parents or the home situation.†

A student experience I count as almost wholly positive was a summer spent with the Henry Street Visiting Nurse Agency in New York City. There I began to discard the formal approach to patients approved in the general hospital. In fact, I acquired a skepticism of medical care in hospitals that remains with me. Seeing the sick return to their homes following hospitalization, I began to realize that the seemingly successful institutional regimen often failed to change the patient's way of living that sent him to the hospital in the first place.

Because nursing in homes seemed so much more satisfying than hospital nursing, I became a visiting nurse after graduation. Several years later I left this field unwillingly to teach in a hospital school of nursing because I was made to feel that the need for instructors was so great. With no special preparation I was forced to learn as I taught in all areas of the curriculum. Over a five-year period I was the only nurse employed to teach in this institution. Fortunately for all concerned, I sensed my need for more knowledge and clarification of my ideas, and I went back to school.

---

* In this era head nurses in many hospitals were, as I have noted, likely to be second- or third-year students.

† It was interesting to find Dr. Veronica B. Tizza of this hospital reporting in 1956 that during the preceding ten years there had been a change of attitude which resulted in a visiting policy that encouraged daily visiting, and that there was an experimental living-in unit for parents.

Except for a brief period of clinical supervision and teaching in a basic university program, I remained at Teachers College, Columbia University, first as a student and then as a teacher, for twenty years. My concept of nursing during this period was not so much changed as clarified. It is impossible to identify all the persons and experiences that brought this about, but the following should be mentioned.

Caroline Stackpole based her teaching of physiology on Claude Bernard's dictum that health depends upon keeping the lymph constant around the cell. This emphasis on the unit structure taught me relationships in laws of health that, to me, had been unrelated up to that time. Miss Stackpole was a master teacher who was never satisfied until the student answered his own question. Jean Broadhurst, a microbiologist, had this same concept of teaching. From them, and through experimentation in the physiology course for medical students of the College of Physicians and Surgeons at Columbia University, I acquired an analytical approach to all aspects of care and treatment. This is more than justified by the articles and books by doctors who are now writing on pathology due to treatment (iatrogenic conditions).[32] As I read reports of malnutrition from therapeutic diets, emotional and physiological crises from endocrine therapy, drug-induced skin lesions, and the varied complications from cortisone administration, I think to myself, "The constancy of the intercellular fluids has been dangerously reduced." Ever since I grasped this danger, I have believed that a definition of nursing should imply an appreciation of the principle of physiological balance. It has made so vivid to me the importance of forcing fluids, of feeding the comatose in some way, or of relieving oxygen want. It was obvious that emotional balance is inseparable from physiological balance once I realized that an emotion is actually our interpretation of cellular response to fluctuations in the chemical composition of the intercellular fluids which produce muscle tension, changes in heart and respiratory rate, and other reactions. Mind and body have come to be inseparable in my thinking. Through this study of physiology the way was paved for acceptance of psychosomatic medicine and all its implications for nursing. In order to understand physical and emotional balance, it has ever since seemed to me to be necessary to start with cell physiology. The man and the amoeba are points on a continuum.*

At Teachers College Dr. Edward Thorndike's work in psychology provided some generalizations, or fixed points, in the psychosocial realm parallel to those I had acquired in the biological sciences. His investigations on the *fundamental needs of man,* including his research into how we spend our money and time, made me realize that illness was more than a state of dis-ease and a threat to life. Too often it places a person in a setting where shelter from the elements is almost the only fundamental need that is fully met. In most hospitals the patient cannot eat as he wishes; his freedom of movement is curtailed; his privacy is invaded; he is put to bed in strange nightclothes that make him feel as unattractive as a punished child; he is separated from the objects of his affection; he is deprived of almost every diversion in his normal day, deprived of work, and reduced to dependence on persons who are often younger than he is, and sometimes less intelligent and courteous.

From the time I saw hospitalization in this light I have questioned every routine nursing procedure or restriction that is in conflict with the individual's fundamental need for shelter,

---

* Just so does Pierre Teilhard de Chardin, the Jesuit priest and scientist, in his *The Phenomenon of Man,* insist on the kinship of *all* matter, going beyond the cell back to the atom. He traces the first manifestations of life to the moment of "revolution" when on the surface of the earth the "biosphere"—or a layer of living cells—formed that new arrangement of molecules having, for the first time, the elusive principle we call "life." His theory, if I interpret it correctly, is a welcome antidote to cynicism. He sees in all matter a movement toward a higher, more complex, or perfect, arrangement of the elements of which it is composed. This universal quality establishes for him man's kinship not only with animals but with what we call inanimate things. His theory demanded of him a humility and universal sympathy that helps, I think, explain the piercing beauty of his countenance. It may be that future generations of scientists will find in the study of atoms a far greater enlightenment than past generations have experienced in the study of cells. de Chardin, Pierre Teilhard: *The Phenomenon of Man.* Harper and Brothers, New York, 1959, p. 318.

food, communication with others, and the company of those he loves, for opportunity to win approval, to dominate and be dominated, to learn, to work, to play, and to worship. In other words, I have since conceived it to be the aim of nursing to keep the individual's day as normal as possible—to keep him in "the stream of life" to the extent that it is consistent with the physician's therapeutic plan.

If for too long we deprive a person of what he values most—love, approval, fruitful occupation—this condition of deprivation is often worse than the disease we are attempting to cure. If a person did not fear this complete dislocation of his life—this yawning abyss between himself and the healthy— sickness and even old age would lose many of their terrors.

Soon after this enlightenment I saw the work of Dr. George G. Deaver and the physical therapists associated with him at the Institute for the Crippled and Disabled and later at Bellevue Hospital, both in New York City. In these programs I found the implementation of many ideas I had been accumulating.[33, 34] I noted that much of the effort of the expert in rehabilitation went into building the patient's independence—the independence of which hospital personnel had unwittingly deprived him or had failed, at least, to encourage. Nothing has made my concept of nursing more concrete than the demonstrations and writings of these rehabilitation experts with their insistence on individualized programs and constant evaluation of the patient's needs and his progress toward the goal of independence. I believe the 1937 revision of the National League of Nursing Education's basic curriculum guide reflected these ideas and that ever since they have been part of the profession's lip service, if not its actual service, to the sick and disabled.[35]

Figure 1 makes the aim of rehabilitation concrete. It shows a list of the activities in daily living. Opposite are spaces in which members of the medical team record the patient's progress toward independence in the performance of these activities. After seeing this form in use, the goal behind it, for me, has been interwoven in the fabric of nursing.

INSTITUTION *Community Rehabilitation Center*

DAILY ACTIVITY RECORD OF

BY MARY ELEANOR BROWN

This Daily Activity Record is for a disabled person of any age who has motion difficulties of any origin hampering everyday living.

Its purpose is to serve as a basis for a rehabilitation program by providing a record of daily activity achievement.

It follows the disabled person through his medical and education periods until he has reached the height of his progress from bed to job.

These Record Blank Forms:
Supplied by Eastern New York Orthopedic Hospital-School, Inc., 124 Rosa Road, Schenectady 8, New York.
Instructions for Use:
"Daily Activity Inventory and Progress Record for Those with Atypical Movement," by M. E. Brown. In The American Journal of Occupational Therapy, beginning with Vol. IV., No. 5, September-October, 1950. (Reprints available: M. E. Brown, 124 Rosa Road, Schenectady 8, New York.)

COPYRIGHT 1950 BY MARY ELEANOR BROWN

RECORD OF: *Doe, John, Jr.*
INVENTORY DATE (5): *1/9/48*
TOTAL TIME: *1 hr. 30 min.*
EXAMINER'S SIGNATURE: *Ellen Diller*

(6) GRAPH KEY

INVENTORY		
WITHIN TIME	BLACK	
WITHIN TWICE TIME	BLACK	
NOT WITHIN TIME OR TWICE TIME		
NOT APPLICABLE		

PROGRESS			
WITHIN TIME	RED	DATE	
WITHIN TWICE TIME	RED	DATE	
WITHIN TWICE TIME, LATER WITHIN TIME	BLACK	RED	DATE
WITHIN TWICE TIME, LATER WITHIN TIME	RED	RED	DATE

(11) SCORES

1/9/–8	2/14/48	3/14/48
54	61	68
1st	2nd	3rd

4/15,–8	5/15/48	6/23/48
92	97	100
4th	5th	6th

(1) CLASSIFICATION	(2) INVENTORY LIST	(3) TIME ALLOWANCE	(4) NO.	(5) GRAPH	(7) SYMBOL	(8) TIME	(9) DATE	(10) NOTES
XII. TRAVELING, UPRIGHT	Public vehicles, upright.	Traffic	100	red		not timed	6/23/48	
	Crossing dummy street on green light, upright.	22"	99	red		22"	6/9/48	
	Floor to standing.	1'	98	red		10"	5/19/48	This tires him greatly
	Standing to floor.	1'	97	red		4"	5/12/48	
	Automobile to standing.	1'	96	red		28"	4/7/48	
IV. DRESSING & UNDRESSING	Putting on and adjusting necktie.	1'	25		ON			
	Fastening shoes or tying shoestrings.	1'	24			24"		
	Dressing except for fastening shoes or tying shoestrings and putting on and adjusting necktie.	15'	23		DRESS	7'40"		
III. BATHING & GROOMING	Shaving or applying cosmetics—(motions).	30"	22			30"		
	Washing body—(motions).	30"	21		WASH	30"		
	Brushing teeth—(motions).	30"	20			30"		
	Combing hair—(motions).	30"	19			30"		
	Cleansing after bedpan use, bed—(motions).	10"	18			10"		
	Off bedpan, bed.	30"	17		OFF	4"		
TOILET, BED	On bedpan, bed.	30"	16	red		57¼"	2/10/48	This is hard to learn Patience
	Readjusting clothing as if after bedpan use, bed.	30"	15		CLO	11"		
	Adjusting clothing as if for bedpan use, bed.	30"	14		CLO	10"		
	Urinal, bed—(motions).	10"	13			10"		
	Sitting to lying (not falling), bed.	10"	12			7"		
	Lying to sitting, bed.	30"	11	red		54", 15"	2/10/48	Comes up slowly one week
II. BED	Edge to edge, bed.	30"	10			5"		
	Left side to back, bed-lying.	20"	9		L B	1"		
	Abdomen to left side, bed-lying.	20"	8		A L	2"		
	Left side to abdomen, bed-lying.	20"	7		L A	3"		
	Back to left side, bed-lying.	20"	6		B L	2"		
	Right side to back, bed-lying.	20"	5	red	R B	1"	1/13/48	
	Abdomen to right side, bed-lying.	20"	4		A R	2"		
	Right side to abdomen, bed-lying.	20"	3		R A	3"		
	Back to right side, bed-lying.	20"	2		B R	1"		
I. SPEECH	Speech.	10"	1			10"		
CLASSIFICATION (1)	INVENTORY LIST (2)	TIME ALLOWANCE (3)	NO. (4)	GRAPH (5)	SYMBOL (7)	TIME (8)	DATE (9)	NOTES (10)

FIGURE 1. Record of daily activities prepared for handicapped persons during the period of rehabilitation. (Brown, Mary E.: "Daily Activity Inventory and Progress Record for Those with Atypical Movement," *Am. J. Occup. Therap.*, 4:195 [Sept.] 1950)

My participation in preparing the 1937 *Curriculum Guide*, in the work of the NLNE's special committee on postgraduate clinical courses, and in the regional conferences associated with Miss Brown's study forced me to express in writing these evolving concepts of nursing.[36, 37] It was not until the 1940s, however, that I could test my ideas in actual practice. It was then that we developed at Teachers College what was, at the time, a unique type of advanced study in medical-surgical nursing.

This course was unique because it was patient-centered and organized around major nursing problems rather than medical diagnoses and diseases of body systems. Related field experience gave the graduate nurse student an opportunity to increase her competence, for example, in helping a patient, and sometimes his family, to cope with a chronic condition; to help him prepare for, and recover from, surgical procedures; to help him to deal with a communicable disease that necessitates relative isolation, or with depression after the loss of a breast or a leg. It was one of the first advanced clinical courses that required students to actually nurse patients under a case assignment system and to conduct nursing clinics and interprofessional conferences around the care of the patients they nursed. The emphasis was on comprehensive care and, to the extent that hospital regulations permitted it, we were concerned with follow-up care.

Associated with me in planning or teaching, or both, were Margaret Adams, Marion Cleveland, Ruth Gilbert, Marguerite Kakosh, Katherine Nelson, Frances Reiter (Kreuter), and Jean South. Exchanging views with these clinically able nurses and with students who were often experienced and expert, I gained immeasurably. When in the fifties I revised the Fourth Edition of Bertha Harmer's and my text *The Principles and Practice of Nursing,* I could present what seemed to me a tested and specific definition of nursing.

Since that time the writings of psychiatric nurses, particularly those of Gwen Tudor (Will) and Ida Orlando (Pelletier), have made me realize how easily the nurse can act on misconceptions of the patient's needs if she does not check her interpretation of them with him.[38, 39]

At the Yale University School of Nursing, where Miss Orlando was when she wrote *The Dynamic Nurse-Patient Relationship,* the faculty stated in 1959 this tentative definition of nursing: "The nurse's prime function is to enable the patients to utilize health measures which are available or prescribed."[40] The principal aim of teaching and research within this graduate program is "systematic study of the nature and effect of nursing practice." Most, if not all, members of this faculty believe that the analysis of the nurse's clinical experience, the identification of the effect on the patient of what she does, is the way to develop nursing theory, generalizations, or guidelines for action. Ida Orlando's book is a series of partial case histories around which she relates examples of patient behavior, as the nurse observes it, the nurse's related thoughts and feelings which she may share with the patient in her effort to get at the true meaning of the patient's facial expression, what he says or how he acts. Miss Orlando describes what the nurse does to meet the patient's need for help after he has confirmed her interpretation of his need, and how the nurse judges her effectiveness by whether the patient's need for help was met.

Ernestine Wiedenbach further clarifies this deliberative nursing process in her monograph *Clinical Nursing: A Helping Art.*[41] She also stresses the point that a worker's goal influences the way he or she works and that how the nurse functions depends upon her philosophy. Here I would like to make the point that these books and the numerous published reports of the Yale faculty and students reinforce Miss Orlando's conclusion that the most effective nursing involves continuous observation and interpretation of patient behavior, validation by the patient of the nurse's interpretation of his need for help, and action based on this validated inference.[42] Faculty discussions and study of their published and unpublished writings have contributed to my present concept of nursing. Faye Abdellah's study of the covert or concealed problems of the patient is related to the concepts just discussed, as is Helene Fitzgerald's work with Yale University students.[43, 44] Unfortunately, it is impossible to mention all the nurses whose works have influenced my thinking.

In 1958 I was asked by the Nursing Service Committee of the International Council of Nurses to prepare a small pamphlet on basic nursing. I quote from this pamphlet, published by the Council in 1961, the following definition of nursing. It is an adaptation of the statement in my last revision of Bertha Harmer's text and represents the crystallization of my ideas:

The unique function of the nurse is to assist the individual, sick or well, in the performance of those activities contributing to health or its recovery (or to peaceful death) that he would perform unaided if he had the necessary strength, will or knowledge. And to do this in such a way as to help him gain independence as rapidly as possible. This aspect of her work, this part of her function, she initiates and controls; of this she is master. In addition she helps the patient to carry out the therapeutic plan as initiated by the physician. She also, as a member of a medical team, helps other members, as they in turn help her, to plan and carry out the total program whether it be for the improvement of health, or the recovery from illness or support in death. No one of the team should make such heavy demands on another member that any one of them is unable to perform his or her unique function. Nor should any member of the medical team be diverted by non-medical activities such as cleaning, clerking, and filing, as long as his or her special task must be neglected. All members of the team should consider the person (patient) served as the central figure, and should realize that primarily they are all "assisting" him. If the patient does not understand, accept, and participate in the program planned with and for him, the effort of the medical team is largely wasted. The sooner the person can care for himself, find health information, or even carry out prescribed treatments, the better off he is.

This concept of the nurse as a substitute for what the patient lacks to make him "complete," "whole," or "independent,"

by the lack of physical strength, will, or knowledge, may seem
limited to some. The more one thinks about it, however, the
more complex the nurse's function as so defined proves to be.
Think how rare is "completeness," or "wholeness," of mind and
body: to what extent good health is a matter of heredity, to what
extent it is acquired, is controversial, but it is generally admitted that intelligence and education tend to parallel health
status. If then each man finds "good health" a difficult goal, how
much more difficult is it for the nurse to help him reach it: she
must, in a sense, get "inside the skin" of each of her patients in
order to know what he needs. She is temporarily the conscious-
ness of the unconscious, the love of life for the suicidal, the leg
of the amputee, the eyes of the newly blind, a means of locomo-
tion for the infant, knowledge and confidence for the young
mother, the "mouthpiece" for those too weak or withdrawn to
speak, and so on.[45]

It is my contention that the nurse is, and should be legally,
an independent practitioner and able to make independent
judgments as long as he, or she, is not diagnosing, prescribing
treatment for disease, or making a prognosis, for these are the
physician's functions. But the nurse is the authority on basic
nursing care. Perhaps I should explain that by basic nursing
care I mean helping the patient with the following activities
or providing conditions under which he can perform them
unaided:

1. Breathe normally.
2. Eat and drink adequately.
3. Eliminate body wastes.
4. Move and maintain desirable postures.
5. Sleep and rest.
6. Select suitable clothes—dress and undress.
7. Maintain body temperature within normal range by adjusting clothing and modifying the environment.
8. Keep the body clean and well groomed and protect the
   integument.

9. Avoid dangers in the environment and avoid injuring others.
10. Communicate with others in expressing emotions, needs, fears, or opinions.
11. Worship according to one's faith.
12. Work in such a way that there is a sense of accomplishment.
13. Play or participate in various forms of recreation.
14. Learn, discover, or satisfy the curiosity that leads to normal development and health and use the available health facilities.*

In helping the patient with these activities the nurse has infinite need for knowledge of the biological and social sciences and skills based on them. There are few more difficult arts than that of keeping a patient well nourished and his mouth healthy during a long comatose period, or that of helping the depressed, mute, psychotic individual re-establish normal human relations. No worker but the nurse can and will devote himself or herself consistently day and night to these ends. In fact, of all medical services nursing is the only one that might be called continuous.

This unique function of the nurse I see as a complex service. A Canadian physician, whose name escapes me, said there are two essentials: care (by the nurse) and cure (by the physician). He added, "I do not know which is nobler." Lord Horder, an English physician, speaks of nursing as a part of medicine.[46] Dr. William R. Houston, late author of *The Art of Treatment,* points out that in some conditions nursing care is the only

* It is my belief that this list of activities can be used in evaluating nursing. In other words the extent to which nurses help patients acquire independence in performing these functions is a measure of their success. Where independence is unattainable, evaluation may be based on the extent to which the nurse helps the patient accept his limitations or his death, when this is inevitable. No effort is made here to describe the way in which the nurse helps the patient with these daily activities. This is done briefly in the ICN pamphlet and more fully in *Textbook of the Principles and Practice of Nursing,* 5th ed.

known therapy. He devoted a section of his text to patients who are to be "treated chiefly by nursing care."[47]•

In emphasizing this basic, or unique, function of the nurse, I do not mean to disregard her therapeutic role. She is, in most situations, the patient's prime helper in carrying out the physician's prescriptions, and her very relationship with the patient can be itself therapeutic.

If we put total health and medical care in the form of a pie graph, we might assign wedges of different sizes to members of what we now refer to as "the team." It is, however, my contention that in some situations certain members of the team have no part of the pie, and the wedge must differ in size for each member according to the problem facing the patient, his ability to help himself, and whoever is available to help him. The patient and his family *always have a slice,* although that of the motherless newborn infant in a hospital nursery or the unconscious hospitalized adult are only slivers. In such cases the patient's very life depends on hospital personnel, but most particularly on the nurse. In contrast, when an otherwise healthy youth is suffering from a skin condition such as acne, he and his physician might compose the team, and they might divide the pie between them. When a patient is ambulatory with an orthopedic disability, the largest slice may go to the physical therapist or, in certain stages of adjustment to an amputation, to those who make and fit prostheses. When a sick child is cared for at home by the mother, or if we admit the mother to the hospital with the child, her share may be by far the largest. But of all members of the team, excepting the patient and the physician, the nurse has most often a piece of the

---

• Lydia E. Hall reports an experience at the Solomon and Betty Loeb Center at Montefiore Hospital, New York City, which illustrates this point. Patients are admitted to this unit because they need nursing care primarily. Physicians are called in by the nursing staff as the need for the services arises. Nursing is recognized as the main line of therapy. Hall, Lydia E.: *Project Report. The Solomon and Betty Loeb Center at Montefiore Hospital.* The Center, New York, 1960, p. 80.

pie, and next to theirs I believe hers is usually the largest share. Figures 2, 3, and 4 show conditions in which nurses play minor and major roles. Figure 5 shows how, with the same patient, the nurse plays a major role in one period and gradually assumes a diminishing role as other workers take over and as the patient acquires independence.

In talking about nursing we tend to stress promotion of health and prevention and cure of disease. We rarely speak of the inevitable end of life and what the nurse might do to help a person reduce its physical discomforts—to face death courageously, with dignity, and even bring to it an awesome beauty.

Anthropologists and other critics of our European culture say we are prone to shrink from the thought and sight of old age and death. In fact, we exalt youth, hiding the signs of age in ourselves as long as possible. In this country, when the aged person loses his independence, we are likely to tuck him away in a nursing home. It is poorly named for it has few characteristics of a home and there is little nursing, as I describe it here. Such custodial care as the average nursing home offers is a national disgrace.

For those who did not hear her speak when she was in the United States, I'd like to mention Cecily Saunders and her work in a London hospital.[48, 49, 50] Possibly because she is a nurse and a social worker, as well as a physician, she has developed a remarkable system of terminal care for cancer patients. Her institution provides an environment that appears to be cheerful and otherwise pleasing to the senses. More particularly she has learned to give those who face death emotional support and to control pain without producing coma, agitation, or the personality changes seen with drug addiction. She shows one photograph after another of a person eating a meal, sitting in a chair in the ward or on the terrace, knitting, or occupied with a game, and she says, not without pride, that he or she died three days later, or "He died peacefully the next day." After she spoke to a large audience of medical students, physicians, and nurses in

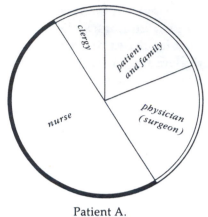

Patient A.

Rational adult first day after operation for cataract in hospital.

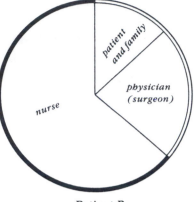

Patient B.

Comatose adult in hospital after surgery for skull fracture with brain damage.

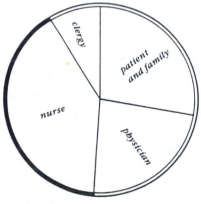

Patient C.

Hospitalized school-age girl with acute cardiac failure.

Patient D.

Motherless hospitalized newborn infant, father unknown.

FIGURE 2. Conditions in which the nurse plays a major role.

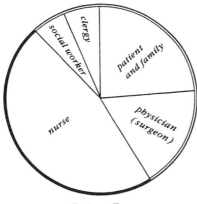

Patient E.

Mature rational hospitalized woman in body cast.

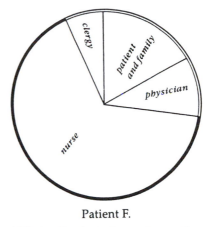

Patient F.

Elderly disoriented man in nursing home.

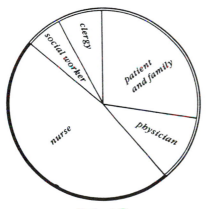

Patient G.

Depressed unwed mother living alone. Referred to VNA by psychiatric clinic where patient fails to keep appointments.

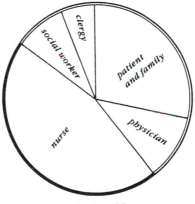

Patient H.

One-year-old baby with no diagnosed disease. Referred to VNA because he "fails to thrive."

FIGURE 3. Conditions in which the nurse plays a major role.

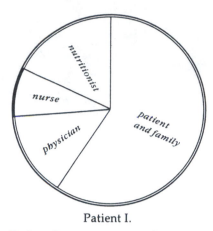

Patient I.

Rational young man under treatment for obesity in clinic.

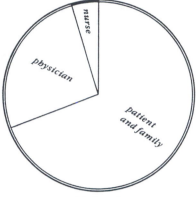

Patient J.

Rational adolescent girl under treatment for acne in a doctor's office

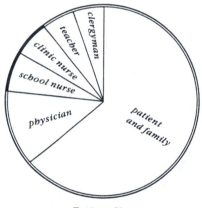

Patient K.

Disturbed 10-year-old boy under treatment in a mental health clinic.

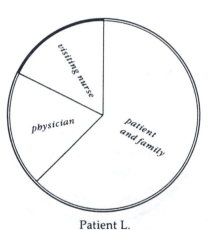

Patient L.

Normal newborn infant girl delivered in home with living parents and siblings.

FIGURE 4. Conditions in which the nurse plays a minor role (assuming that all other persons contributing to patient care are available).

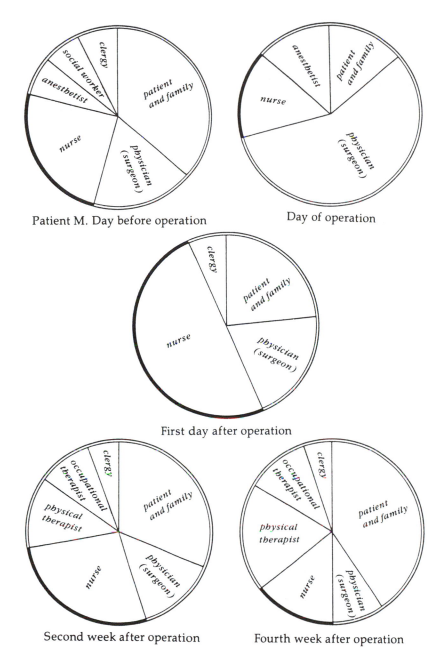

Patient M. Day before operation

Day of operation

First day after operation

Second week after operation

Fourth week after operation

FIGURE 5. Showing how the nurse's role diminishes as rehabilitation progresses in the case of a young man having a leg amputated, for example.

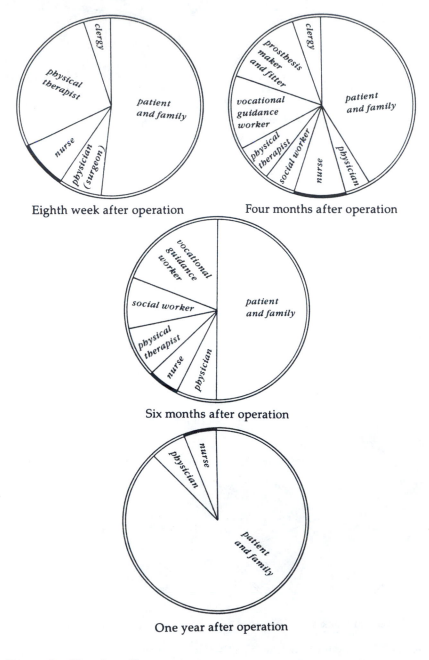

Eighth week after operation

Four months after operation

Six months after operation

One year after operation

FIGURE 5. *(Continued)*

30

New Haven, Dr. Saunders had a standing ovation.* It would be too bad if the competences of the nurse and the physician must be literally embodied in one person to bring about their full engagement in the improvement of terminal care. But with or without prescriptions from the physician that reduce pain and coma to a minimum, the nurse can still do a great deal anywhere to keep the environment in which death occurs supportive and esthetic; she can reduce the patient's discomfort with nursing measures and reduce his loneliness in death by facing it with him honestly and courageously. If the nurse has a religious belief akin to the patient's, she can reinforce his faith; but in any event she can see that he has the help he wants and needs from the minister of his choice.

In summary, I see nursing as primarily complementing the patient by supplying what he needs in knowledge, will, or strength to perform his daily activities and to carry out the treatment prescribed for him by the physician.

---

* Dr. Saunders always attributes to other members of the hospital staff, but particularly those of the religious nursing order there, much of the credit for patients seeming to feel safe, or at peace.

ADDENDUM
DEVELOPMENT OF A PERSONAL CONCEPT

The nature of medical treatment has changed so greatly since 1966, and the technology employed by doctors *and* nurses has developed so rapidly, that my personal concept would undoubtedly reflect some aspects of those changes were I writing about health services today. Treatment has not only become more complex technically but, in this country, far more costly. This is especially true of hospital services, which has resulted in their being reduced in length with more and more emphasis put on home care.

The cost of nursing care—and all health care—has increased so much that it overrides other considerations. While I may not be informed enough to comment on this, I believe that the ownership of hospitals affects this practice. A hospital operated to make money operates differently from one that is not influenced by the financial return but rather by the therapeutic results for which it is known.

In the United States more than 12 percent of the gross national product is spent on health care. This expenditure is not the rule elsewhere in the world. Japan, for example, spends roughly half the U.S. amount and has better statistics for longevity, maternal and infant health, and deaths from heart disease than the United States can claim.

The United States is often cited as the only industrialized country, with the possible exception of South Africa, that has no universally available tax-supported health insurance. Medicare and Medicaid, which were created to provide for the needs of the elderly and the indigent, have both been so misused that they partially fail to meet their respective aims.

Military personnel, and governmental employees generally, have tax-supported health care. When speaking or writing about health care today, I leave no doubt in the audience's mind that I think this should be universal. In 1966 I was not so aware of how peculiar the United States was in regard to providing all its citizens with the essential elements of health care. I now believe that without increasingly available tax-supported health care nurses will find it impossible to provide the care implied in my "personal concept." If writing today, I would put more emphasis on universally available care and on the preparation of citizens to assess their need for help and to help themselves effectively. I would stress that health care is a *political* subject.

Today I see the role of nurses as givers of "primary health care," as those who diagnose and treat when a doctor is unavailable, even as the midwife functions in the absence of an obstetrician. Nurses may be the general (medical) practitioners of tomorrow. Because of that, I also emphasize the extent to which not only doctors and nurses but all health care personnel *share* responsibility for providing care, particularly in underserved areas.

Writing today, I put more stress than I did in 1966 on the health record and the roles of health care consumers and providers in making and using it. I would advocate every one having, as military personnel have, a personal copy of his or her health record. A lengthy medical record can now be put on a single microchip which can be kept with other essential records.

While I made no reference in 1966 to the role of the nurse in helping people have "a good death" when death is inevitable, I would now put more emphasis on the question of prolonging life beyond the period of its usefulness. The importance of working with families and the patient over issues of "the right to die" or dying with dignity are increasingly a part of nursing care. The development of hospices and the kind of terminal care they typify has affected the concept of the care of dying patients in all institutions and settings and certainly reflects a change since 1966.

3

Implications for Practice

*T*he nurse who sees herself as reinforcing the patient when he lacks will, knowledge, or strength will make an effort to know him, understand him, "get inside his skin," as I have said. This process of putting oneself in another's place is always difficult and only relatively successful. It requires a listening ear and constant observation and interpretation of nonverbal behavior. It also demands of the nurse self-understanding and the recognition of emotions that block her concentration on the patient's need and helpful responses to these needs. It calls for a willingness on the nurse's part to selectively express what she is feeling and thinking so that a *mutual* understanding may develop between nurse and patient.

The nurse who tries to put herself in the patient's boots can use unlimited knowledge of the general laws underlying human behavior and specific knowledge of peoples, in different cultures and walks of life. Miss Goodrich thought the latter knowledge part of being "socially experienced," and she attached great importance to it.

The practitioner implied in the definition of nursing discussed here will not take at face value everything a patient says. He or she will realize, for example, that few persons give a truthful answer to the question, "How do you feel?" If they doubt the questioner's sincere interest, they say "very well," "all right," or "fine" because this closes the conversation. The nurse who genuinely puts herself in the patient's position, who wants to know and has reason to doubt the accuracy of such a statement, says "What do you mean 'very well'—you look uncomfortable to me." One patient in answer to this comment said, "To tell you the truth, I do feel all right *physically,* but I'm *mad* because I can't get a cup of hot coffee in this hospital!" A trivial matter such as this is easy to handle, and it was relatively simple to satisfy the patient's wants. Another incident illustrates the more serious consequences of assuming that the patient will express his needs, fears, and anxieties without a special effort by medical personnel to convince him of their interest and readiness to help him: A young man after a surgical operation appeared to have a remarkably uneventful recovery. The young nurse who presented him with considerable pride in a nursing clinic commented on it. But the patient said, "You didn't know what I was thinking the morning after my operation; that was bravado! No one told me I would be put in a room beside the nursing office instead of in the open ward where I had been before the operation. I suffered torment all night thinking I had been put there because I was dying. I was not really reading the *New Yorker*—I was just holding it in front of my face." In this case the wrong could not be redressed. The nursing staff had lost its opportunity to get at the true meaning of a patient's behavior and to give him the help he needed.

Volumes have been written on the process of developing empathy or a helping relationship with another human being. Psychoanalysts, who rely on this for successful practice, have influenced medical literature as a whole and much of our current fiction. The stream-of-consciousness novel is an attempt to contrast what the person is thinking with what he is doing.* Counselors of the Carl Rogers School make use of a variety of techniques to get at the unexpressed and subconscious motivations of behavior.

I am not suggesting that nurses should be psychoanalysts or guidance experts. I do believe, however, that great medical and nurse practitioners through the ages, either deliberately or intuitively, have used some of the methods that our current psychotherapists have developed into a system. But nurses of this age are fortunate in having made available to them this systematized knowledge of man's nature.

In a brief work such as this, it is impossible to develop any topic in detail. However, I can suggest that the reader will profit by studying the descriptions by nurses of the analytical, "deliberative," approach which is designed to help the nurse understand the patient. Florence Burnett's and Maurice Greenhill's writings are one example.[51] I have called attention to Faye Abdellah's study of the covert or hidden problems of patients and to Gwen Tudor Will's detailed reporting of successful intervention of the nurse where there had been mutual withdrawal of patient and medical personnel. I have stressed as especially applicable to all nursing the accounts by Ida Orlando (Pelletier) and Ernestine Wiedenbach of the interactions of patients and nurses. They give specifically in each case what the nurse observes, what she thinks or feels, what she says or does in response to this thought or feeling, and how the patient responds, how he affirms or denies the nurse's interpretation of his problem or his needs, and finally how the nurse evaluates her success in helping the patient to solve his problem or meet his need.

The nurse who wants to understand and help each patient will welcome opportunities to see and talk with his friends and family. In some cases it is important to observe an adult at

---

* Cecil Woodham Smith's biography of Florence Nightingale is of great interest partly because she made full use of her subject's notes to herself. In it we learn how Florence Nightingale saw herself as well as how others saw her. In these notes she reveals herself.

work or a child in school. If the cause of his illness is to be known, if his independence is to be established and a recurrence prevented, the nurse who participates in all these aspects of comprehensive care must work with and through others. *Her greatest contribution may be to help a member of the family to understand what the patient needs from him or her.*

No matter what the setting, the nurse who is reinforcing, or supplementing, the patient will help him perform all the functions enumerated on page 22. She will make with the patient, his family (if it is involved), and other members of the health team some sort of individualized plan, or daily regimen, that meets the wide range of human needs. She will not be satisfied to see provided only the bare essentials of shelter, sanitary facilities, three meals a day, and treatments prescribed by the physician. Figure 6 is an example of such a daily plan.* In addition a long-term plan will be made, ideally by the health team, the patient, and the family.

Although the nurse seeks to help the patient meet his needs during a period of dependency, she also tries to shorten this period. Before she carries out any act for him, she asks herself what part of it he could himself perform. If he is unable to act at all, she tries to identify what he lacks and to help him develop, as rapidly as possible, the necessary will, strength, or knowledge required for the act.

In other words the rehabilitation of all patients in the hands of such a nurse begins with her first service to him. With this point of view, and if she has a wide range of competence, the

---

* Gladys Nite and Frank N. Willis, in their study *The Coronary Patient: Hospital Care and Rehabilitation* (New York, The Macmillan Co., 1964), show a series of individualized plans that take into account a full range of patient's needs during hospitalization. Some nurses object to any written plan as suggesting rigidity—failure to provide for the immediate and changing needs of the patient. If the plan is not subject to continuous revision, it can have this undesirable effect. However, I contend that with rare exceptions everyone has, and needs, a pattern or design for living in health and in sickness. Although it should provide primarily for the person's needs, realistically it also must be fitted into the pattern of living in the community of which he is a part.

PLAN OF CARE

NAME _Hamilton, Mrs. Esther_   DIVISION _C Medical_   HISTORY NUMBER _856,239_

HOUR	DATE 6-2-65 2 3 4 5 6 7 8	TREATMENT AND NURSING CARE	SUGGESTIONS FOR GIVING CARE
AM 7:00	+ + + + + + + +	On high-low bed, alternating pressure mattress. Elastic stockings. Record intake (2500 ml. minimum) and output. Positive pressure mask (10 min.) Offer bedpan (Skin care)	Speech slow, with some aphasia. Can write with left hand. Do not hurry speech or motion. Accept Mrs. Hamilton's depression and emotional responses. Encourage her to question and express fears and desires. Give realistic encouragement.
8:00	+ + + + + + + + + + + +	T.P.R. and blood pressure Face and hands bathed Arms and legs - range of motion Mouth cleaned. Fluid 2 glasses Breakfast (Regular diet)	Rectal thermometer seems to cause discomfort. Insert with special care, well lubricated (Patient will exercise unaffected arm and leg.) Have patient in sitting position when eating and drinking to avoid insufflation. Encourage drinking before breakfast to stimulate defecation reflex afterwards. See that
9:00	+ + + + + + + +	λ Alpha-E Succinate, 200 I.U. Colace 240 mg. Encourage bowel movement in toilet - Commode wheel chair Shower in wheel chair	food is prepared so that it can be eaten with one hand. Support in chair with hip and shoulder belts Stay in bathroom with patient. Is afraid of straining since hemorrhage occurred during defecation Give bed bath if patient is too tired for shower
10:00		Rest in bed (horizontal)	Going by clocked sign, or record, at bedside help into alternate positions in bed — supine, lateral, prone, supine, lateral, prone etc. Use pillows to support, abduct and elevate arm, handpad to prevent finger flexion, trochanter roll to prevent thigh abduction, foot board or sand bags
11:00	+ + + + + +	Offer bedpan (Skin care) Positive pressure mask (10 min.) Encourage coughing To Physical Therapy Department Rest in bed (horizontal) on return	to prevent foot drop. Keep heels free of mattress. Put on plastic pants with absorbent liner under day-clothes before taking to Physical Therapy Department. Use sling on unaffected arm.
12:00	+ + + +	Refer to Speech Clinic and Family Health Service. With them Mrs. Hamilton and her family work out plan for home care. Blood pressure	Husband, daughter and special friend (Mrs. Archer) visit patient daily. Accept their help and teach them as much as possible as a means of preparing Mrs. Hamilton and family for her return home
PM 1:00	+ + + + + +	Luncheon, sitting up in bed or in wheel chair Mouth cleaned Offer bedpan (Skin care)	Encourage (family) visitors at lunch time. As she improves suggest to Mrs. Hamilton that she have meals with ambulatory patients in dining room. Stress fluid intake while sitting up. Help patient to assume responsibility for drinking and for recording intake
2:00	+ + + +	Rest in bed (horizontal) always alternating positions	Induce sleep, if possible, with quiet, cool and darkened room. See that feet are warm. Put sign on door "Sleeping." (Mrs. Hamilton is distressed by disorder in room. Daughter tells us she has always avoided signs and odors of illness in the home)
. 3:00	+ - + + +	Offer bedpan (Skin care) To Physical Therapy Department if tolerated	Plastic pants etc., as above Keep diaprene impregnated incontinent pads on bed under buttocks and use wide draw sheet protection.
4:00	+ + + + +	Rest in bed (horizontal) on return Positive pressure mask (10 min.) Encourage coughing	
5:00	+ + - + +	Offer bedpan (skin care) Up in chair if tolerated T.P.R. and blood pressure	As Mrs. Hamilton improves can be rolled out into garden where grandchildren can pay her brief visits
6:00	+ +	Dinner sitting up in bed or in wheel chair	Encourage fluid intake up to 10 P.M. to avoid necessity of drinking latter part of night.

| NAME | Hamilton, Mrs Esther | DIVISION | C Medical | HISTORY NUMBER | 856.239 |

HOUR	DATE 6-2-65 2 3 4 5 6 7 8	TREATMENT AND NURSING CARE	SUGGESTIONS FOR GIVING CARE
PM	+ + + + + +	1 Alpha-E Succinate 200 I.U. Colace 240 mg. 1 multivitamin capsule	As bowel movements get normal, or can be regulated with diet, fluids, position and regimen reduce dosage and finally omit Colace
7:00			
	+ + - + +	Offer bedpan (Skin care) Up in chair, as tolerated Blood pressure	Family may read to patient, or, if she has no visitors encourage to look at television in sitting room, or listen to radio
8:00	+ +		
	+ +	Positive pressure mask (10 min.) Encourage coughing. Prune juice and crackers	Check fluid intake and encourage drinking as indicated Mrs. Hamilton is accustomed to bedtime "snack"
9:00	+ +		
	+ + + +	Offer bedpan Evening toilet - Back bathed and rubbed. Use silicone lotion, baby powder or A and D ointment according to condition of skin on buttocks	Encourage sleep with quiet, cool and darkened
10:00			
	+ +	Change elastic stockings powder feet	room. Be sure feet are warm
11:00			
12:00	+ + + +	Offer bedpan (Skin care) Blood pressure	
AM			Encourage sleep etc. as above Do not wake for care during remainder of night but if Mrs. Hamilton is wakeful or restless offer bedpan, change position and exercise arms and legs at intervals
1:00			
2:00			
3:00			
4:00			
5:00			
6:00			

FIGURE 6. Plan of care for Mrs. Esther Hamilton, a 59-year-old librarian employed in a large urban center. The patient lives with her husband, a retired university professor. A daughter and her family live nearby; a married son is in Europe. Now, in the third week of her illness following a cerebral hemorrhage, Mrs. Hamilton's prognosis is good, although she has a weakness of the right arm and leg and some speech impairment.

nurse can be the prime rehabilitative agent.* Such a nurse judges her success with each patient according to the speed with which, or the degree to which, he performs independently the activities that make, for him, a normal day.

This primary function of the practicing nurse, of course, must be performed in such a way that it promotes the physician's therapeutic plan. That means helping the patient carry out prescribed treatments or administering the treatment herself. Again, she will consider herself more successful if she assists the patient or motivates him to independent action.

During periods of prostration or of coma and irreversible illness, when dependence and death are believed inevitable, the nurse's goal changes. She remains, under such conditions, indispensable. Her object then, as I implied earlier, is to protect the patient from loss of dignity during this period of inescapable dependence. The nurse will be alert to what gives the patient physical and spiritual comfort and will seek out for him the persons he needs, if this is possible, and will do what she can to see that they are not barred from his presence. I have discussed the care of the dying patient in Chapter 35 of *Textbook of the Principles and Practice of Nursing.*[52] It is inappropriate to go into further detail, except to say that the writings of Cecily Saunders, referred to earlier, especially have increased my understanding of the needs of patients with intractable pain. Although prescribing narcotics is wholly within the physician's realm, the handling of his p.r.n. directions can make the difference between relative comfort for the patient and an insatiable need for the drug in question. For this reason Dr. Saunders doubts the wisdom of putting the patient in the position in which he fears his pain will not be controlled unless he

---

* To make this concrete I would like to cite an experience in a Veterans Administration hospital for paraplegics. I was taken to one ward to meet a head nurse who was said to be exceptional. I asked in what way and was told that sooner than other head nurses on five similar units with the same medical staff she got the patients to sleep without narcotics, she helped them regain urinary continence, she helped them to be ambulatory rather than bedfast and interested in recreational activities.

demands the drug. In other words, she questions the use of these p.r.n. prescriptions.

The nature of pain and its control deserve study by nurses as well as physiologists, psychologists, and physicians. The nurse who is with the sufferer more constantly than any of these workers has, for this reason, a better opportunity to investigate its clinical aspects. The studies of Anne Bochnak and Julina Rhymes, as two examples, suggest that the nurse with an inquiring mind, a "deliberative" approach, and the earnest desire to help the patient can often identify other needs when the patient complains of pain, which, if met, relieve this state of dis-ease.[53, 54] Too often drugs are used in excess because they are the quickest and simplest means of dulling all sorts of psychological and physical suffering. How to meet intractable pain and death remains in every culture a major concern. The nurse who attempts to identify with every patient under her care is inevitably involved.*

In certain situations the nurse may find it necessary to assume the role of a physician—in hospitals with no medical resident or intern, for instance, or in emergencies. First aid, which has elements of diagnosis and therapy, is expected of all informed citizens under certain conditions. Soldiers are taught to give their wounded comrades infusions, and policemen are expected to deliver a baby if no medically trained person is available.

In hospitals lacking resident medical staffs, in industry, home nursing services, and schools, physicians connected with these services may supply covering directives that delegate medical functions to the nursing staff. Such written statements help, but do not fully protect, those concerned.

As long as nurses are better prepared than any other member of the health team to act as a physician surrogate, they will be

---

* Dorothy M. Crowley at the University of California, Los Angeles, and Bonnie Hoffman at the University of Missouri are other nurses studying the nature of pain and its relief.

tempted, in the interest of the patient, to assume this role. But it is not, in my judgment, their *true role*. In assuming it they not only practice skills for which they are ill-prepared but also rob themselves of the time needed for the performance of their primary role. Inevitably, when nurses take over the physician's role, they delegate their primary function to inadequately prepared personnel. In my opinion, social pressures should promote an increase in the number of doctors (just as social pressures have promoted a phenomenally rapid increase in nurses) so that medical functions need not be delegated.

This brings us to the question of the coordinating, managerial, and teaching functions that now consume so much of the professional nurse's time. Nurses are, of course, appropriate administrators of nursing services and teachers of nursing, but whether they should coordinate the services of the medical team is questionable. I, for one, am glad that experiments such as those at the Memorial Hospital in New York City and at the hospital of the University of Florida in Gainesville are helping to demonstrate the relative advantages and disadvantages of non-nursing coordinators and administrators of clinical units.[55, 56] Dorothy Smith, Dean of the nursing school and *chief of nursing practice* in the Florida center, discusses some of its problems in an article entitled "Myth and Method in Nursing Practice." She emphasizes the importance of developing a system, or an environment, in which the nurse can function as effectively as she knows how to function. She identifies poor communication as one of the prime deterrents to effective patient care and unrealistic goals as a source of frustration for medical personnel. Numerous nurses in this country have insisted that members of the occupation must be freed from all non-nursing tasks and that an environment must be created in which they can function in peer relationships with other professional medical workers. The writings of Dorothy Smith, Thelma Ingles, Florence Flores, Florence R. Weiner, and Frances Reiter Kreuter are some examples.[57, 58, 59, 60, 61]

When we insist, as I have in this booklet, that patient care should be individualized and that the nurse will seek constantly to help the patient meet his needs and live as normally as it is possible for him, I may fail to stress, as I should, that the best nurse under the best circumstances operates within limits, which Dorothy Smith mentions. Family life and institutional, or communal, living imposes limits. The necessity for the nurse to operate as a member of a medical team imposes other limits.

Ernestine Wiedenbach in *Nursing as a Helping Art* discusses this question of the conditions that the nurse may think hamper creative nursing. She points out that the nurse's temperament also imposes a limitation on her performance, and she suggests that there are no easy answers to whether we should accept or refuse to accept the conditions that impose limits. However, she implies that with sufficient self-awareness, we can modify the temperamental barriers, or self-imposed limits, to effective nursing. According to the nurse's philosophy and her concentration on the goal of patient welfare, she will find ways of promoting this goal in spite of conditions in the situation she might like to alter. Nurse readers will find Miss Wiedenbach's philosophical approach to this perennial and personal question interesting and helpful.

Finally, to close the discussion of how my definition affects practice, I point out that the nurse who sees her primary function as a direct service to the patient will find an immediate reward in his progress toward independence through this service. To the extent that her practice offers this reward, she will be satisfied; to the extent that the situation deprives her of it, she will be dissatisfied. And she will use whatever influence she has to foster conditions that make the social rewards for practice at least commensurate with those for teaching and administration.

ADDENDUM
IMPLICATIONS FOR PRACTICE

This addendum applies equally to my concept of nursing and to implications for practice today. My concept implies, if it does not specify, universally available health care. It suggests, if it does not specify, a partnership relationship between doctors, nurses, and other health care providers with patients and their families.

None of these conditions are the rule in the United States although some providers and recipients of care may enjoy them in some situations. Especially is this true in hospices for the terminally ill. Health care is not universally available but beyond the reach of many. The relationship between doctors and the public is not universally helpful, nor is the relationship between doctors and nurses. Doctors rarely teach now in educational programs for nurses. For this and other reasons there are fewer opportunities than there were in earlier years in this country for these two providers of health care to know each other.

However it was a satisfaction to find at the University of Vermont the personification of the helping relationship I would like to see developed everywhere demonstrated by Dr. Lawrence Weed and the other health care providers associated with him. At this Vermont health center an extensive record of the experience and needs of the patient is elicited from the patient with a multiple-choice questionnaire which the patient answers by touching the face of a computer. This information is available to all health care providers who care for or treat the patient at this center. The patient's record is developed as a cooperative effort of the recipient and providers of care and treatment.

This system at the University of Vermont, as it was used at that time, is described in considerable detail in the 1978 revision of the text *The Principles and Practice of Nursing.* Ever since seeing this demonstration of health care delivery at this Vermont center, I have seen it as the kind of care the citizens of this country have a right to expect. Those of us who believe this have no other choice than to work to establish this as a universally available system in its essential aspects.

4

Implications for Research

When a nurse operates under a definition of nursing that specifies an area in which she is pre-eminently qualified, she automatically imposes on herself the responsibility for designing the methods she uses in her area of expertness. Studies of nursing functions, such as the statewide California study, identify more than 400 specific acts performed by hospital nurses.[62] Many of these are non-nursing acts that could be assigned to other personnel; some are medically prescribed procedures for the design of which the physician is, at least, partly responsible. But if the nurse carries out the latter procedures and is liable, in the legal sense, for harmful effects on the patient, she *must* share the responsibility for the design of the procedure with the physician.

Many procedures have to do with care, rather than cure; they do not require a physician's prescription and, in fact, he is relatively unaware of how they are performed. It is my contention that methods in this area will remain static and will become invalidated if the nurse fails to study them. Most aspects of basic nursing, including the nurse's approach to the patient

(what she may and may not say or do for him), are steeped in
tradition and passed on from one generation of nurses to another. Too often they are entrenched routines without rhyme or
reason. They are learned by imitation and taught with little, if
any, reference to underlying sciences. This is amply demonstrated in the study by Julius Roth, "Ritual and Magic in the
Control of Contagion."[63]

Most persons would claim to act reasonably. We act on a
belief we hold at the moment, and this belief represents a fact
to the person holding it. We come to these beliefs through one
or more processes that might be arranged in the following
progression:[64]

1. Intuition (a glimpse of "truth" through unconscious
   effort).
2. Authority, tradition, custom.
3. Chance (accidental personal experience).
4. Trial and error (deliberate personal experience).
5. Generalization from experience.
6. Logic, deduction, syllogistic reasoning, or a formal
   argument with a major and minor premise and a
   conclusion.
7. Inductive reasoning—a conclusion arrived at by related particulars, especially numerous observations.
8. Research, scientific inquiry, or a structured, systematic investigation designed to answer a question, throw
   light on a theory, or solve a problem.

It seems obvious that all these processes are useful, even
necessary. The relative uses and values of each are subjects of
endless debate among poets, priests, philosophers, and scientists. Perhaps the most civilized man is the one who recognizes
all of them and chooses in each case what he believes to be the
appropriate basis for his acts.

If nursing is, to any extent, a science, it must use the method
of inquiry characteristic of it. Research is the most effective
method yet designed for finding unity, order, or relationships

so that we can set reliable guides for conduct. They may not be final; they are subject to revision as further research sheds more light on the question and as creative imaginations see new relationships. In this age all professions and large industries use scientific inquiry in the solution of their problems, as a basis for their programs. Is it not natural for nurses to do likewise?

The difficulty of presenting an argument for research by nurses lies in my inability to see any argument against it. Unless one believes in the "born nurse" or in the assumption that a nurse acts under the orders of the physician who will design the methods she uses, there seems to be no reason why she should not subject her practice to the same type of analysis that characterizes all comparable occupations. Actually, in this country at least, nursing studies multiply so rapidly that their very existence refutes any argument.

Ellwynne Vreeland, reviewing the nursing research programs of the U.S. Public Health Service last year, reported that this agency alone has invested $8,672,700 in 132 projects since 1955.[65] But only in recent years will we find emphasis on research in nursing practice.

In a survey and assessment of nursing research reported in 1964, Leo W. Simmons and I have pointed out the preponderance of educational and occupational studies over clinical investigations.[66] We tried to identify the conditions that discouraged patient-centered research. Those who are interested may consult this report for fuller treatment of the question. Some of the conditions we identified are the following: The major energies of the occupation have gone into improving the preparation for nursing and learning how to recruit and hold sufficient numbers of workers in the occupation to meet the growing demand for service; the need for administrators and teachers has almost exhausted the supply of degree holders, therefore nurses with a university background have tended to study administrative and educational problems; and the few nurse practitioners interested in, and prepared to conduct, research have often failed to get the support they needed from hospital administrators, nursing service administrators, and physicians.

Although physicians usually depend on the help of nurses in clinical research, they rarely regard them as partners. Not too long ago, Dr. Bayne-Jones made the observation that a laboratory technician participating in medical research was more likely to be recognized as a joint author of a report than was a nurse.[67] Doctors may be startled to find that some nurses are initiating and designing investigations of nursing practice. But if, by definition, nursing has an area of independent professional practice, is not clinical nursing research as necessary as clinical medical research? Do we not deny this independent function when we fail to investigate it?

The Surgeon General's Consultant Group on Nursing, in its summary and recommendations says, "Nursing research must be stimulated. Research in nursing has just begun to yield the body of knowledge needed as a basis for the improvement of nursing care. . . . Much greater support than is currently given is required for patient-oriented studies in line with the changing patterns of nursing care."[68]

It is not only in this country that the need for research in nursing practice is recognized. Margaret Jackson, a British physician, has expressed some of these ideas simply and directly:

Research into nursing methods and appliances possibly began with Eve. Miss Nightingale and the generation of nurses trained under her aegis took it, of course, immeasurably further; but since their day it seems to have come to a dead end of evolution, like the frog. The basic techniques of bed-making, blanket-bathing, giving an enema, administering medicines, and the like, seem hardly to have changed within the memory of woman; and few nurses seem to pause and ask themselves whether their methods and equipment are the best possible, or whether in fact they might be better.

The teaching of medical students flourishes in an atmosphere of research. . . . It seems to me that nurses too would be stimulated by working in an atmosphere of research; but

of research into their own specialty, not of medical research
. . . . I believe it is time that nursing research was revived.

For some reason "nursing research" is taken, at present, to
mean those investigations, made mainly by people outside the
profession, into the nursing hours spent on this or that service to
patients—job analyses, in fact. Some studies of course are extremely valuable, but they are not, in my view, nursing research:
that can be done only by nurses actively engaged in nursing, and
in training nurses. There are three broad lines, I suggest, on
which nursing research might develop.

First, I really do think there is scope for improving nursing
practice. . . . The second subject on which I think nursing research is badly needed is the design of nursing equipment.

This talk of measuring brings me to my third suggestion for
nursing research. Many nursing practices produce results which
ought to be measured. Miss Nightingale, who was a pioneer of
statistics, would certainly have approved their use for assessing
the value of nursing techniques. It would be well worth know-
ing, for instance, what proportion of elderly patients come to
their end while struggling on and off a bed-pan; what proportion
of stout elderly patients burst their stitches after operation, and
whether this proportion could be reduced, and their pain less-
ened, by providing them all with a handle on a chain, over the
bed, by which they could pull themselves up to a sitting position; and what is the incidence, and the time of onset, of foot-
drop due to the weight of bedclothes on the feet of patients
confined to bed.

Any experienced nurse could add to this list; and she might
also add that everybody knows the answers without statistics.
That may or may not be so; statistics sometimes produce sur-
prises. But a scientific study backed by figures, might often be
the means of bringing up-to-date measures into the less advanced hospitals. Moreover, it might also strengthen the hand of
a matron who had long been trying to get—say—a better design
of bed-pan, a better type of bed, or enough cradles to prevent
foot-drop in all the patients in her hospital.[69]

It is my belief that every clinical service of a hospital needs a medical research committee and a nursing research committee—both devoted to the ultimate common goal of improving patient care. The medical research committee would study those matters lying wholly in the realm of medical practice; the nursing research committee would investigate questions, procedures, or problems that lie wholly within the realm of nursing practice. But another committee, a joint committee, composed of representatives of the medical research committee and the nursing research committee, is needed to study such treatments or diagnostic tests as are prescribed by the physician and carried out entirely or partly by the nurse. Other specialists such as the microbiologist, physiologist, chemist, psychologist, sociologist, physical therapist, nutritionist, or social worker may be asked to work with any one of these committees as and when the problem involves his field. Figure 7 is a diagram showing such an organizational plan for a hospital. Figure 8 suggests three types of problems that concern the nurse.

The first type of problem has to do with activities the nurse may initiate—those the patient would carry out unaided if he had the will, the strength, and the knowledge. The second type of problem has to do with treatments or tests prescribed by the physician but carried out by the nurse, or the patient and the nurse. The third type of problem is related to treatments or tests prescribed by the physician and carried out by him with minimal nurse participation.

I believe that it is the nurse's responsibility to initiate and conduct research on the first type of problem, with whatever consultative help she may need. I think it is her responsibility as much as the physician's to initiate research on the second type of problem. However, since the physician prescribes the treatment and therefore must be answerable for its effect, research on such measures, even though the nurse carries them out, should involve the physician. Investigations of problems related to treatments and tests performed by the physician with minimal nurse participation should be initiated by the physician and

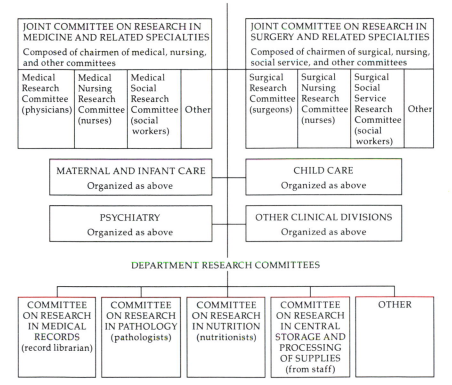

FIGURE 7. Organization within a hospital for study of method in care of patients.

CLASS I. The nurse (or a nursing committee) appropriately investigates any activities she initiates and performs as, for example, the following:

1. Clean the mouth of a bedfast unconscious patient when there are no lesions in the mouth.
2. Keep the intact skin clean and prevent pressure sores in the paraplegic.
3. Move, lift, support, or feed by mouth the physically helpless.
4. Encourage an apprehensive patient to void or micturate.
5. Protect the disoriented or delirious person from bodily harm.
6. Encourage the withdrawn or the psychologically mute to speak.
7. Encourage the patient to express his needs, fear, or anxiety.

CLASS II. The nurse (or a nursing committee) appropriately initiates and investigates, with a physician (or a medical committee) any of the treatments he prescribes, but which she carries out, or helps the patient or his family carry out as, for example, the following:

1. Clean the mouth of a baby following an operation for cleft palate.
2. Dress and promote the healing of a decubitus ulcer.
3. Apply a sling to a fractured arm.
4. Feed an infant through a nasal tube.
5. Operate the drainage device and keep adequate records of intake and output of fluids when a patient has an indwelling urethral catheter.
6. Observe and record the patient's symptoms during a seizure, or convulsion, and respond to him in a protective and therapeutic manner.
7. Use restraining devices with disoriented, assaultive, or self-destructive patients.

CLASS III. The nurse (or a nursing committee) does not initiate, but appropriately works with a physician (or a medical committee) in studying activities or treatments prescribed and carried out by the physician with nurse participation, or in some cases without, as for example, the following:

1. Graft skin.
2. Remove a foreign body from the larynx.
3. Apply a plaster cast.
4. Prepare a patient for taking a general anesthetic.
5. Control intractable pain with drugs.
6. Act on a patient's refusal to accept treatment.
7. Respond to the patient's questions as to whether he is dying.

FIGURE 8. Three classes of problems that concern the nurse, and her relative responsibility for initiating and conducting research on each for validating or improving practice.

conducted largely by medical personnel but with nursing represented on the research team.

Those interested in my analysis of the nurse's responsibility for initiating and participating in research might also want to study David J. Fox's model for identifying research areas in nursing.[70]

Some of the graduate students at Yale, all of whom conduct at least one patient-centered investigation, have been troubled by the accusation they hear or read that nurses are seeking status through the conduct of research. But is this not a criticism leveled at every medical worker?

Dr. Louis Lasagna, in a witty article entitled "Statistics, Sophistication, Sophistry and Sacred Cows" says, "We are all snobs (with apologies to Russell Lynes) of course. The ego, sometimes referred to as a fragile gossamer thing, actually has an omnivorous appetite. It subsists on a diet of favorable comparisons with other egos over which it possesses a real or imagined superiority. Medical research has always provided a bounteous banquet-table for starved egos, but in recent years has begun to nourish in greater numbers persons whom I shall call statistical snobs. . . ."[71] I imagine that similar comments could be found on research in almost every field. It seems to me that we must dismiss as unimportant the risk of being thought a status seeker when we promote research on nursing practice.

For emphasis I repeat that the nurse who operates under a definition that specifies an area of independent practice, or an area of expertness, *must* assume responsibility for identifying problems, for continually validating her function, for improving the methods she uses, and for measuring the effect of nursing care. In this era research is the name we attach to the most reliable type of analysis. It is based on the full use of scientific findings and is the most orderly approach man has invented to the solution of his problems.

As I have attempted to show on page 46, it is only one of the roads we take in our search for truth. We think now that it is our most direct road. It seems to take us nearer our goal than the other roads, but truth, fact, or an absolute, like infinity, seems to be something we approach but never reach. The findings of our best research, after all, must be interpreted by man, and machine deductions are dependent on man's design of the machine and the information he feeds into it. Conclusions based on today's research may be upset by more extensive and improved research in the future. Social scientists question the methods of the physical and medical scientists and vice versa.

Nurses have borrowed methods from the social scientists in studying the nurse-patient relationship—that subtle and fundamental aspect of nursing—and also in evaluating nursing care as based on the satisfaction of patients, nurses, and other medical personnel. Nurse researchers have also used research methods of medical and biological scientists in studying certain aspects of their work.

Some persons believe that nurses must design their own research techniques in order to get at the inwardness of nursing—an analysis of how we reach our stated goal. They suggest that only by this step can we establish nursing as a distinct science different from other medical sciences. Although this is an arresting and challenging idea, it need not stand in the way of our also borrowing research methods and findings from the pure and applied sciences in the improvement of nursing practice. If medicine had not borrowed from physics and chemistry—the more basic sciences—it would never have made its spectacular advances. However, I suggest that those especially interested in the development of nursing theory through research might study the writings of Florence Wald and Robert Leonard,[72] Myrtle Irene Brown,[73] and Katherine K. Kelly and Kenneth R. Hammond.[74]

I conclude that no profession, occupation, or industry in this age can evaluate adequately or improve its practice without research. Readers who are interested in reviewing studies focussed on nursing care might consult Chapter 13 in Leo Simmons' and my report (*Nursing Research; A Survey and Assessment*).

I have quoted Dr. Jackson's plea for developing student nurses in a research atmosphere. Later I will stress the importance of a problem-solving approach to the study of nursing on all levels. Frances C. Macgregor describes convincingly, and in some detail, the "Research Potential of Collegiate Nursing Students."[75] It should be unnecessary to point out that graduate nurses brought up under an authoritarian system must go through a period of "unlearning," or adjustment, before they can adopt the analytical attitude toward nursing implied in the definition discussed in this monograph.

A number of schools in this country offer undergraduate introductory experience in research, some have programs to develop research competence in their faculties, and occasionally we see a building plan for a school of nursing that includes research laboratories. Such signs lead us to hope that the inferences we are drawing are shared by a rapidly growing body within the nursing occupation.

ADDENDUM
IMPLICATIONS FOR RESEARCH

Nursing is widely claimed to be a "research based" occupation. In the preceding discussion, research is identified as one of the eight processes nurses use in arriving at a valid reason for their actions. Research involves time-consuming steps and is not appropriate for making the minute-to-minute decisions that life demands of all of us. Research is no substitute for the instinctive, intuitive reactions we have to situations; however, these instinctive, intuitive reactions are influenced by our knowledge of the sciences that guide human behavior in the society of which we are a part.

Therapists of this age base their practice on psychological and biological research. They try to learn the reason why an agent is effective, and very often they find that therapy is ineffective because the knowledge of the underlying science is inadequate or is wrongly interpreted. Much of nursing practice has been based on custom, or tradition, or the authority that has assumed responsibility for nursing practice.

In this country nurses are now trying to base their practice on the same sort of scientific knowledge that guides other providers of health care. I hope the idea is increasingly dominating nursing that *all* practice demands workers who have the habit of study; who realize that health care *must change* daily in response to research findings; that effective nurses are lifelong students.

My introduction to research in nursing was provided by Martha Ruth Smith when I first went to Teachers College as a student during the 1920s. I was her assistant in teaching an introductory course in research to graduate nurse students from this and foreign countries. When Miss Smith left to direct the nursing program at Boston University, I inherited the courses she taught at Teachers College. Both Miss Smith and I emphasized the application of research to *nursing practice*. Ever since, I have assumed that this emphasis should be encouraged and maintained.

56

With the profession's decision in the early 1950s to stress research, Leo W. Simmons and I were asked to make a survey of existing nursing research. Mr. Simmons was an anthropologist at Yale University, and the grant to finance this survey was given to the School of Nursing at Yale. I went to thirty states asking influential persons in these states what nursing research had been done there, what studies they knew about, and what studies they would conduct if they had the necessary resources.

The information accumulated in this survey indicated that the awareness of research as a means of improving or validating nursing education and practice was extremely limited. Educators, however, were more aware of its value than practitioners. It was also clear that faculty members advising nurses conducting research were from the social rather than the medical sciences. I think this is true to this day.

After Mr. Simmons joined the nursing faculty at Teachers College, I moved from the Graduate School to the Nursing School at Yale. Florence Wald, then its dean, sensed the value of the bibliography I had developed in Mr. Simmons office. She got a grant from the U.S. Public Health Service to prepare this bibliography for publication. An advisory committee for this publication was established, along with a committee to coordinate the work of those agencies concerned with the development of library resources for nursing. The latter group, The Interagency Council on Library Resources for Nursing, exists today and meets twice yearly. It has published bienially in *Nursing Outlook* a list of journals, books, and other sources focused on nursing.

The work at Yale, instigated by Florence Wald, developed into an eleven-year project, culminating in the publication by J. B. Lippincott Company of a four-volume annotated index to the analytical and historical aspects of the English literature on nursing from 1900 through 1959. The production of this index and the promotional efforts of the Interagency Council on Library Resources in Nursing resulted in the creation of the *International Nursing Index* in 1966, published quarterly by the *American Journal of Nursing* in collaboration with the National Library of

Medicine in Bethesda, Maryland, which also publishes the *Index Medicus*.

All the experience outlined above has prepared me to see research in nursing as *essential* to the validation and improvement of practice. In recent years schools of nursing have added to their faculties one or more persons prepared to teach the research method. These persons have usually been social scientists. They have not only taught the process of research but have been advisors to nurse students conducting research. This has resulted, perhaps, in undue emphasis on social rather than medical problems. Research collaboration of nurses and therapists (doctors) has not been encouraged.

If I were writing *The Nature of Nursing* today, I would include enough history of the development and practice of research by nurses to enable them to understand why it has developed as it has—why the research has not been more focused on the practice of nursing. Attending a conference on research in nursing recently, I was encouraged by its concentration on problems in practice—on the care of the elderly and, for example, on the prevention of falls and the control of incontinence.

What may have been interpreted in recent years as the technology of medicine has resulted in a counter-revolution in nursing, manifested as an emphasis on *caring*. I would leave no doubt in the reader's mind that I believe caring for those they serve is an important, really essential element of nurses' service. I would try to describe or discuss nursing in such a way as to convince the reader that nursing practice and nursing education should nevertheless be based on research.

5

Implications for Nursing Education

A definition staking out an area of health and human welfare in which the nurse is an expert and independent practitioner calls for education rather than training. This kind of nursing demands a liberalizing education, a grounding in the physical, biological, and social sciences, and ability to use analytical processes. In my opinion it implies certain conditions within the organizational structure of the school; it suggests policies underlying faculty appointment and student selection; it demands certain facilities and resources; it influences curriculum and teaching methods.

The following suggestions are offered to those who find the concept of nursing expressed in this booklet reasonable and who have every right to say "How would you go about teaching it?" I can offer only an outline or a framework. I have myself used some of these ideas in the education of basic and graduate nurse students, and I have seen many of them adapted to a variety of programs by graduate students with whom I have worked.

59

The ideas apply, in my opinion, to all types of programs in this country. Certain principles are applicable to nursing education in any country.

Organizational Structure of the School

There may be many organizational plans under which a successful school can operate, but some conditions seem to me essential. One is that the students have an opportunity to see and to practice a high quality of nursing care, and the other is that the school function as an educational institution.

There is a Chinese saying—"I forget what I hear, I remember what I see, I know what I do." Only the most creative and imaginative students will learn how to give patient-centered, family-centered, or comprehensive care if they never see it given or participate in it. I believe that those educators who are trying most earnestly and successfully to teach effective nursing are themselves demonstrating it.

This statement, if true, suggests a reorganization of many schools and nursing services of hospitals and other field agencies. It implies that teachers must be able to influence the quality of nursing service. The educator who holds a joint appointment in the school and the nursing service is in the best position to establish an environment in which she and her students can practice nursing as the school defines it. Liaison committees, frequent conferences, and other means of promoting understanding between educators and service personnel are, of course, important, but the educator is in a stronger position when he or she can effect changes in practice by direct executive action rather than through an indirect approach.

Clinical instructors function most effectively if they are assigned to a small enough unit to enable them to know the patients; otherwise they cannot give students the kind of help they need in working with patient's problems. Since patient turnover, the type of service, and other conditions affect the number of patients the instructor can know, it is difficult to say what the ratio of patients and students to instructor should be. In the past we generally have erred in assigning such large services to clinical faculty members that they have been unable to successfully help students meet the individual needs of patients. Whatever the ratio, I suggest that the organizational plan should provide students with tutorial clinical guidance from those who have the knowledge and the authority to help them (the students) effect a solution of nursing problems. This seems to me the most important administrative policy to stress in the present era.

It is generally accepted, and need hardly be stressed here, that learners should have student status, and that although nursing students may give service in order to acquire the knowledge, skill, and judgment expected of graduate nurses, they should not be exploited. This is particularly what is meant by the statement that the school should be organized to operate as an educational institution and not as a training program in a service agency. However, there are many other reasons why those learning to nurse should have the same benefits of student status enjoyed by those learning comparable arts and sciences.

Student Selection

It seems obvious that what we can teach the students in a nursing program of any given length depends to a great extent on the students' intelligence, character, physical fitness, educational background, and social experience—in other words, on what they bring to it. Naturally one can expect of college graduates a more mature understanding of man, his fundamental needs, his motivations, and the way he responds to life situations than one can expect of high school graduates. The desire for self-knowledge, for good relationships with others, and for learning how to be good parents often leads college students to take many of the science courses on which a clinical nursing curriculum is built—physiology, psychology, human development, anthropology, and sociology. If they are especially interested in science, they may study, in addition, physics and chemistry, or possibly microbiology.

The student of nursing cannot acquire a systematic knowledge of human behavior and development, of group behavior, and of therapeutics without constant recourse to the physical, biological, and social sciences. If these sciences are not prerequisites, they must be given before the clinical instruction begins or concurrently with it; or the needed science must be woven into the clinical program.

Although I believe that all these patterns can produce effective nurses, it seems to me self-evident that the ease and rapidity with which nursing students can be prepared depends, other things being equal, on their having had a liberal education with a high science content.

Mark Van Doren in his study *Liberal Education* concluded that it should enable its possessor to recognize what is common to all men and to be equally sensitive to their differences.[76] Clearly these abilities are of paramount interest to nurses. We want to provide for man's universal needs but with infinite modifications in nursing care according to the ever unique requirements of the individual. Therefore, the nurse educator can but rejoice when the student brings with her this feeling of the oneness of mankind and the sensitivity prompting him or her to treat each person as unique.

Incidentally it is said that those who write fiction or biography capture our interest in their human subjects to the extent that they describe each person's *peculiar,* or *distinctive,* characteristics. It may be that knowledge of the general with application to the specific is central to artistic performances in all arts—including the art of nursing. A great deal more can be said about the selection of students, but these observations must suffice. The use of tests, interviews, and other devices for assessing attitudes and personality, important as they are, must be left unexplored in this booklet.

Choice of Clinical Faculty

In discussing the organizational plan that my definition implies, and in other connections, I have indicated that those who teach nursing must practice it, and that each instructor should function on a unit that is small enough for her to know all the patients with whose problems she and her students will be concerned.

A school influenced by the definition under discussion therefore will select clinically expert nurses as instructors. If the students profit by having a liberal education and a strong science background, this is equally true for instructors. In addition, they will be most effective if they have had post–basic preparation in their chosen clinical field. If, on the other hand, medical and health services come to be organized according to the amount of care the patient requires, as in intensive- and self-care units, the special preparation sought among the faculty may change in nature. Whatever the change may be, the principle is the same—that the clinical faculty should be expert in practice (as the school defines it), able to analyze and evaluate nursing activity, at ease in the clinical teaching situation, and able to give to students the help they need in acquiring clinical competence.

While clinical nursing instructors should carry the major responsibility for teaching, many other staff members can and should contribute. Comprehensive medical care requires cooperation, understanding, and mutual esteem among many kinds of medical workers, for example, physicians, nurses, social workers, physical therapists, occupational therapists, nutritionists, clinical psychologists, and other social scientists. All should have some appreciation of the others' roles. If the student is to learn to work as a member of this team, she must have this appreciation of everyone else's function. Most especially, if she is to help the patient carry out the prescribed therapy, she must have considerable knowledge of medicine.

Because physicians have not always adjusted their teaching to the needs of the student nurse, the tendency in recent years has been to limit their role in the school of nursing. In my judgment there is no substitute for the discussion of therapy by the therapist. I believe nurses must learn medicine from the physician. (And by the same token, the medical student must learn nursing from the nurse if he is prepared to be an effective member of the team helping the patient.)

If, in teaching diagnosis, pathology, and therapy, the physician focusses on a particular patient, his contribution will never lack interest and meaning for the undergraduate or graduate student nurse. Physicians who can and will teach with this focus make an invaluable contribution to nursing education.

Medical teaching is enhanced in most cases by group teaching in which other members of the health team discuss that aspect of the patient's care for which they are responsible. In this way the student acquires a feeling for the whole program, the difference in the roles of medical workers, and how they complement each other. Students will also learn in group teaching sessions how the contribution of the physician, nurse, religious counselor, social worker, or physical therapist varies according to the nature and phase of the illness (see Figure 5). For example, when a person is dying, the minister may be able to give the patient more comfort than any other member of the health team; but when a person is recuperating from an illness that is limiting his body function, a vocational guidance worker who can help him find suitable employment may be, at one point, his chief helper.

Finally, among those who may be counted as teachers of clinical nursing, the patient has more to contribute to the nurse's education than anyone else *if she can learn to let him show her what help he needs*. Also, patients who have made a good adjustment to a condition that, as Dr. Houston says, "limits living," for example, a leg amputation, a colostomy, gout, or diabetes, can often contribute to the education of the entire medical team and to the rehabilitation of other patients with the same condition. Some of the most helpful group teaching sessions we had in an advanced medical-surgical nursing course were those in which a former patient was a member of the teaching panel. In some cases we brought in members of the family, and they likewise were helpful.

In summary I might say that all types of personnel who serve the patient directly can contribute to the student nurse's understanding of, and ability to participate in, comprehensive medical care.

Facilities and Resources

The concept of nursing that is the central theme of this volume implies that the nurse is a generalist. The school that accepts this definition therefore will feel obligated to give the student experience in the care of patients of all ages and in all major services. At present, we think of the latter as medicine and surgery (with their related specialties), maternal and child health services, and psychiatry. The concept I am attempting to implement also implies that nurses are able to care for people through all phases of illness and in normal states, such as infancy and pregnancy, that require the help of nurses or their substitutes.

If the ultimate goal of nursing is the person's independence and prevention of lapses into dependence, nursing must have continuity. It is difficult or impossible to offer students an opportunity to see and participate in all phases of rehabilitative and preventive health care within the hospital. Experience in other health agencies and in home care programs therefore is indicated until, and unless, hospitals are reorganized to be health centers that give total health service in a given locality. It is conceivable that they will be and that all types of health personnel will eventually move freely from the hospital or health center into convalescent units, clinics, homes, schools, or industries in order to provide optimum continuity of care.

If the emphasis in nursing education is on developing the students' ability to supplement the patient in carrying out his daily regimen and the physician's prescribed therapy, she must acquire first of all the ability to develop this helping relationship with the patient. If this help is individualized, the care of each patient presents a unique problem, and the student must develop analytical powers and problem-solving techniques; no routine can be learned and applied without modification. I believe that the student can acquire this basic helping relationship on any service. However, the most fundamental patient problems vary with age, with the length of the illness, and whether the disease is infectious or associated with unconsciousness and many other factors (see Figure 9). Therefore the clinical facilities and resources should present the student with the opportunity to meet these and other major nursing problems or situations.

Since the definition of the nurse's function implies that she must be able to help the patient with his specific therapy as prescribed by the physician, a knowledge of many conditions and therapies is essential to nursing competence. In other words, the most effective nurse knows a great deal about the art and science of medical practice.

In the past we put great stress on having the student carry out a given list of procedures and having her nurse a given list of diagnoses. At the present time, in an effort to stress the human relations aspects of nursing, as opposed to the technical, we are wont to belittle the value of manual skills and experience in the care of patients with a wide variety of diseases and conditions.

It is my opinion that although the development of the helping relationship and the problem-solving approach to nursing are essential and can be learned in small medical units, the advantage of large medical centers with their richness of clinical experience should not be underrated.

Students who have not participated in the care of patients from such groupings as brain or eye surgery, acute infectious diseases, acute nutritional disorders, or drug addiction are not as well-prepared after they graduate to function in relation to

1. Breathe normally.
2. Eat and drink adequately.
3. Eliminate by all avenues of elimination.
4. Move and maintain desirable posture (walking, sitting, lying, and changing from one to the other).
5. Sleep and rest.
6. Select suitable clothing, dress and undress.
7. Maintain body temperature within normal range by adjusting clothing and modifying the environment.
8. Keep the body clean and well groomed and protect the integument.
9. Avoid dangers in the environment and avoid injuring others.
10. Communicate with others in expressing emotions, needs, fears, questions, and ideas.
11. Worship according to his faith.
12. Work at something that provides a sense of accomplishment.
13. Play, or participate in various forms of recreation.
14. Learn, discover, or satisfy the curiosity that leads to "normal" development and health.

> This includes making a plan for such assistance, taking into consideration the following factors always present that affect the person's needs.

1. Age: newborn, child, youth, adult, middle-aged, aged, and dying.
2. Temperament, emotional state, or passing mood:
    a. "normal" or
    b. euphoric and hyperactive:
    c. anxious, fearful, agitated, or hysterical or
    d. depressed and hypoactive.
3. Social or cultural status:
   A member of a family unit with friends and status or a person relatively alone and/or maladjusted, destitute.
4. Physical and intellectual capacity:
    a. normal weight;
    b. underweight;
    c. overweight;
    d. normal mentality;
    e. subnormal mentality;
    f. gifted mentality;
    g. normal sense of hearing, sight, equilibrium, and touch;
    h. loss of special sense;
    i. normal motor power;
    j. loss of motor power.

FIGURE 9. **Nursing I. Basic Nursing Care.** *Student's major goal:* To acquire competence in helping a person perform the functions listed above or in providing conditions that will enable him to perform them.

patients suffering with these conditions as are students who have had such experiences.

Also, the development of inquiring minds and problem-solving techniques—or a research attitude—demands laboratory and library resources of a quality rarely found in small hospitals. It is particularly important that the student develop the habit of studying each patient's disease or condition while she is caring for him. If she makes a thorough study, it requires access to medical literature and the indexes, abstracts, reviews, and other tools that conserve the student's time. Few small hospitals and their associated nursing schools, even when the hospital and school library are combined, offer the resources nursing students need. If the student is to acquire the ability as a graduate to continually increase her clinical competence, she should begin to practice independent study as an undergraduate.

Improved equipment and numerous and well-furnished practice laboratories facilitate clinical teaching throughout the curriculum. With adequate laboratories it should be possible for students, acting as subjects for each other's practice, to experience many of the nursing procedures and treatments they carry out on patients, from the simplest, such as a shampoo in bed, to living in a respirator. Nursing laboratories and conference rooms on, or connected with, the clinical units facilitate teaching around a patient. He can come to a nursing clinic, for example, if the room is nearby, whereas it may be difficult or impossible to bring a patient to a classroom in a nurses' residence. Clinical classrooms also facilitate the student's practice with bulky equipment such as an oxygen tent or monitoring units. The practice of putting classrooms in residences, I believe, has retarded the development of effective clinical instruction. (Those interested in current thought on nursing education facilities in this country will want to consult the report of the Joint Committee of the National League for Nursing and the U.S. Public Health Service.[77])

Obviously the student's clinical experience can be greatly enriched by observation of, or participation in, health programs in the community, other than those in the main hospital or hospitals with which the school is affiliated. The variety of such experience that it is possible to offer depends on the length of the program and the area's resources. But, in my judgment, the effort to provide variety should not jeopardize the student's opportunity to see and give uninterrupted care of the patients to whom she is assigned. In other words a limited *thorough* experience has more value than a wide range of superficial experience.

On every service the facilities should provide an opportunity to nurse the patient from the beginning of his illness through rehabilitation and the steps taken to prevent recurrence. In my judgment, this is the single most important opportunity the school should offer.

Curriculum, Content, and Design

If the nurse is primarily an independent practitioner rather than coordinator, administrator, teacher, or doctor's assistant, the professional aspects of the curriculum should be organized around her major function rather than that of the physician, as it has been in the past. Emphasis on diseases and defects of body systems with the attendant minutiae of diagnoses and therapies is unsuited to the nursing curriculum. Actually, Dr. William Houston thought the grouping of diseases around body systems the wrong approach to teaching medicine. In his *Art of Treatment* he recommended grouping diseases around the physician's major problem—determining the main form of therapy, as for example, administration of specifics, psychotherapy, limitations of living, and nursing care. He called attention to the fallacy of grouping for teaching purposes a tumor of the lung with a deviated nasal septum or pharyngitis, even though each is a disease or defect of the respiratory tract.[78] In certain medical schools where the faculty is trying to develop a patient-centered, or family-centered, approach to medicine, students begin by studying in the home the psychological and physiological problems associated with pregnancy. From such experiences they identify the knowledge and skills they need and seek help from various sources in the school.

Some educators believe that a curriculum should arise entirely out of the day-by-day experience of the student. Some think that the students should do what planning there is as they feel the need for help in caring for particular patients. Such educators would reduce preplanning to a minimum. This is a rebellion against the traditional system of presenting the student with a logical organization of subject matter, or theory, and expecting her to make the application days, weeks, months, or maybe years later as the need for it arises in practice on the clinical service.

There is no question in my mind that students should participate in curriculum planning and that the essence of good teaching is the development of inquiring minds and the ability to use problem-solving techniques. However, unless each generation is to start from scratch, there must be a *system* of passing on the fruits of experience. For the sake of exposing the greatest number of students to whatever of value the teachers have to offer, we must provide for group instruction as well as for tutorial help.

Group teaching necessitates planning and scheduling. Systems of accreditation and licensure are based, in part, on the guarantee that nursing programs have met certain minimum standards with respect to organized content, including group instruction and field experience. Hopefully we will continue to experiment in nursing education with various curricula as well as with methods of teaching, including the use of all sorts of audiovisual aids and teaching machines.

Nursing literature abounds in reports of educational experiments. The variety of nursing personnel prepared under the different curricula must amaze those who are just beginning to study the occupation of nursing. It is tempting to digress and review some of the more important reports, but such a review is inappropriate in this discussion. I would like, however, to suggest that the reader interested in this brief work study one monograph, *Patient-Centered Approaches to Nursing* by Faye Abdellah, Irene L. Beland, Almeda Martin, and Ruth V. Matheney.[79] All these authors accept as a guide to practice and curriculum building a list of twenty-one nursing problems.* They also describe, in varying detail, a two-year associate degree program, a three-year basic diploma program, and a four-year bachelor of science program—all patient-centered.

Although their twenty-one nursing problems and mine (shown on page 72, Fig.10) differ, there are some similarities. We both emphasize the study of the patient and the individualization of care. Almeda Martin makes the point that we cannot teach everything the student might like to know, but that we can create an atmosphere conducive to learning and can help her develop the habit of study which, if continued as a graduate, will lead to ever-increasing nursing competence.

The clinical curriculum suggested by Figures 9, 10, and 11 shows three stages of learning in which the student progresses from the more universal to the more specific. But the focus in all stages remains the same—supplementing the patient when he needs strength, will, or knowledge in performing his daily activities or in carrying out prescribed therapy with the goal of ultimate independence or rehabilitation, when this is possible.

Figure 9 outlines the content of the first nursing course. It is organized around the fundamental needs of man, planning nursing care, and the nurse's unique function of helping the patient carry out his daily activities or regimen. It takes into account the conditions always present that affect his basic needs, but it does not emphasize pathological states or specific illnesses.

Students study the underlying theory or related science background through class instruction. The related skills, or the

* Olga Andruskiw and Betsy L. B. Battick amplify the material in this monograph by identifying diseases and conditions in which oxygen want and electrolyte imbalance (two of the twenty-one nursing problems) occur ("Identification of Nursing Problems," *Nurs. Res.,* 13:75–76, Winter 1964).

1. Marked disturbance of intake and output of gases demanding medical intervention such as administration of oxygen.

2. Marked disturbance of nutrition, fluid and electrolyte balance, starvation, obesity, pernicious vomiting, diarrhea.

3. Marked disturbance of elimination with constipation, suppression or retention of urine, incontinence of urine or feces.

4. Motor disturbance limiting motion; also prescribed immobilization.

5. Hyperactivity, with or without convulsions or hysteria.

6. Fainting, dizziness (loss of equilibrium), transitory and prolonged coma, or unconsciousness, disorientation, delirium.

7. Insomnia, anxiety, depression.

8. Hyperemia or hyporemia as a result of exposure to environmental temperatures or as prescribed treatment.

9. Local injury, or wound, with infection.

10. A systemic infection, a communicable condition transmitted by various channels, with or without febrile states.

11. Shock, or collapse, with or without hemorrhage.

12. Disorders of communication attributable to congenital defects of sight, hearing, or speech (including deafness and mutism), and such handicaps when imposed by illness or treatment.

13. Preoperative state.

14. Postoperative state.

15. Persistent, or intractable pain.

16. Dying state.

FIGURE 10. **Nursing II. Symptomatic Nursing, or Common Problems in Nursing.** *Student's major goal:* To acquire competence in helping a person carry out prescribed therapy and his daily activities as modified by the symptoms, syndromes, or states (common to many diagnoses) listed above that are encountered by nurses in many settings.

ON MEDICAL SERVICES	
Therapy related to general conditions such as: Long-term illness Metabolic disorders Endocrine disorders Functional disorders Neoplasms Infections Degenerative processes	Therapy related to specific diseases such as: Arthritis Osteomalacia Addison's disease Anemia Leukemia Tuberculosis Cardiovascular diseases

ON SURGICAL SERVICES	
Therapy related to general conditions such as: Preoperative, operative, and postoperative state in Area of surgery { Head and neck Chest Abdomen Pelvis Extremities	Therapy related to specific diseases such as: Brain tumor removal Thyroidectomy Lobectomy (lung) Colostomy Nephrectomy Reduction and fixation of fracture of an extremity

ON MATERNAL AND CHILD CARE SERVICES*	
Therapy related to general states such as: Prenatal Natal Postnatal Newborn Infancy Preschool children Middle childhood Adolescence	Therapy related to specific diseases such as: Eclampsia Caesarean birth Mastitis Erythroblastosis fetalis Eczema Cerebral palsy Poliomyelitis Rheumatic fever

ON NEUROPSYCHIATRIC SERVICES	
Therapy related to general conditions such as: Mental deficiency Pathological personality development Anxiety states—psychoneuroses Acute depression with suicidal tendencies Maniacal states Paranoid states	Therapy related to specific diseases such as: Hydrocephalus Alcoholism and drug addiction Manic-depressive psychoses Schizophrenia

*Another unit might follow this organized around the special needs and diseases characteristic of young adults, middle age, and old age; or such content may be incorporated into units of Nursing I, II, and III and suggested therein.

FIGURE 11. **Nursing III. Disease-Oriented Nursing; Mother, Infant, and Child Care.** *Student's major goal:* To acquire competence in helping a person carry out prescribed therapy and daily activities as indicated by specific diseases and in conditions, or physiological states, such as those listed above.

art of implementing the theory, I suggest they will acquire best through observation of patient care by expert practitioners, through observation of laboratory demonstrations, and through their own practice in the laboratory and in the clinical unit. Students are assigned to patients with experienced nurses who work with them and help them develop an increasing competence. The student is first the participant observer. Later she assumes the dominant role, and the instructor assumes the less active function. Finally, the student, with a safe minimum competence, functions independently in giving these basic aspects of nursing care.

In my judgment students could be assigned to any of the clinical services while they are studying the components of basic nursing. Patients to whom students are assigned should be carefully chosen with consideration for the needs of both. If the clinical instructor knows the patient and the student and is able to teach on a tutorial basis, she can reduce to a minimum the anxiety of the learner and the subject. Whenever a patient is embarrassed or harmed in any way during the learning process, the student has been exposed to a poor example of nursing practice. The learner should never be made to feel that his interests are put before the patient's welfare. This protection both of the student and of the person on whom he or she is learning to nurse calls for instructors who are not only technically able but also skilled in human relationships.

During this first phase of the clinical curriculum, no emphasis is placed on the patient's diagnosis and the physician's plan of therapy, although the student should be helped to learn something about both, if for no other reason than that she will want to know. But at this stage more experienced students or graduates should be giving medications and other treatments. The beginning student should be a junior participant in patient care, giving him limited, but ever-increasing, help.

It seems to me that the first course should be planned and conducted by all the clinical instructors who give tutorial assistance to students on the clinical services. They might appoint a chairman, or the chairmanship might rotate. Specialists should be asked to contribute to the course as needed. For example, a dentist or a dental hygienist might help to teach mouth care; a psychiatrist might discuss theories of sleep and the significance of sleep patterns; occupational and recreational therapists would present some principles and modalities in their field; and a clergyman could explain the significance of the sacraments or dietary laws and other aspects of religions that present problems for patients and personnel during illness and hospitalization.

In some cases the handling of a topic is enriched by group teaching; in others it is wasteful. But group planning is necessary to prevent repetition and omission of important theory and practice.

During this first phase of the clinical curriculum, students who may have had limited experience in helping other human beings find themselves cast in a critical role; people as old as their parents and grandparents, seeing them in uniform, expect skilled service. Many techniques must be learned in a brief period, and, at present, the ability to work effectively with a hierarchy must be acquired if they are to succeed. All studies of student nurses so far show that they work under considerable stress. Their chief source of satisfaction lies in the student-patient relation. This is rewarding and their focus of interest throughout. In my opinion this first phase of the clinical curriculum, like the second and third, should be based in the clinical units. But, for both the student's and the patient's protection, a higher ratio of time should be given laboratory practice than in the second and third phases. Some of this practice should be directed by instructors, but slow learners or those less dexterous manually should be encouraged to spend additional time in the laboratory practicing skills and working with equipment. Laboratories should be considered, like libraries, a place to learn, and insofar as it is possible, both should be open to students during the normal work week.

At the end of this first phase of the clinical curriculum we might expect the student to be able to make a plan for a patient that would include the basic components of nursing and that would help him with the fourteen functions listed in Figure 9. We would expect her to take into account, and be informed about, the modifying conditions of age, temperament, social status, and physical and intellectual capacity. We would also expect her to demonstrate some skill in recording and assessing interactions between herself and her patients.

The second phase of the clinical curriculum is shown in Figure 10. At this time the emphasis is on helping patients to meet their momentary, hourly, or daily needs during marked body disturbances or pathological states that, in themselves, regardless of the disease diagnosis, demand specific responses from the nurse or certain modifications in nursing care. Twenty such states are listed in Figure 10, but experience might show that other states should be included. Most of them occur on every clinical service, but some are seen in the average hospital only on a surgical service, a psychiatric service, or possibly an emergency unit. In order to participate in the care of patients presenting all these problems, therefore, it may be necessary for the student to have experience in a number of clinical services. Patients to whom students are assigned during this second phase are selected for a more specific purpose than in the first phase of the curriculum. The presenting nursing problem is one of greater complexity. More medical science is involved, and the student begins a serious study of the rationale of symptomatic treatment so that she can effectively help the patient to carry out the physician's prescriptions.

Obviously many of the patients to whom the student is assigned in this phase are seriously ill. Needless to say, the student is still a junior member of the team of nurses caring for the patient. She is first an observer, then a participant under guidance, and then she is allowed to function independently when she has demonstrated a safe minimum of competence.

It is my opinion that this second aspect of the clinical curriculum, like the first, should be taught by all the clinical instructors who are giving students tutorial assistance on the various clinical services. Again, the chairman of the course may be appointed or elected, or the chairmanship may rotate. One instructor may be the best prepared person in the group to present principles underlying the care of the incontinent patient, another the disoriented, the depressed, or still another the care of the patient who has a local injury. If a panel of clinical instructors teaches such a course, they may capitalize on the special competence of its members. For a thorough development of a course based on these problems, it is necessary to involve many types of workers, for example, physicians, surgeons, psychologists, physiologists, microbiologists, special therapists, social workers, clergymen, and even technicians who are specially trained to operate the complicated machines that students must now learn to use. These topics may be treated superficially or in depth. Problems such as insomnia, blindness, or intractable pain challenge the graduate and the basic student alike. The research on pain alone fills volumes, and it would take years to read everything that has been written on stress or anxiety. A nursing faculty, therefore, is faced with the necessity of making arbitrary decisions as to how much time can be devoted to these problems. The decision will depend, to a great extent, on the length of the program and the background and interests of the students.

If we are correct in assuming that these are relatively common problems, no student should graduate from a basic program without having participated in helping patients cope with them. Instruction built around them constitutes part of a common core of nursing that cuts across all clinical services as they are now organized. This second phase of the clinical curriculum may be taught concurrently with the third phase or it may precede it.

The third phase of the clinical program is shown in Figure 11. In this phase the focus is on the particular problems the patient faces because he has arthritis, asthma, leukemia, poliomyelitis, a lung tumor, or an acute depression. The list of ills man is heir to stretches on and on. Ideally a general basic program would give students of medicine and nursing an opportunity to help patients with all the conditions they may encounter after graduation; obviously this is impossible.

Many attempts have been made to select diseases and conditions that student nurses *must* know something about—either by observing or by nursing patients with the diseases or conditions. Such lists may be found in published curricula and in student records used in various schools. In my judgment we can help solve this problem by identifying *types* of disease, stressing the pathological processes involved and the rationale of treatment underlying the type, or class, and selecting for special study from this type or class certain of the more common diseases or conditions. I share with many nurse educators the belief that a thorough knowledge of a few conditions is likely to produce, ultimately, a more effective nurse than a superficial knowledge of many.

At this point the student should be acquiring the ability to make a complete patient study. In addition to the more basic nurse competences she acquired in the first and second phases of the curriculum, she will add the total range of competences demanded by the patient's particular condition or illness. The medical science content of the clinical nursing curriculum in this third phase is unlimited. In other words only time, resources, and the student's ability limit what she can profitably learn about the diagnosis, prognosis, and treatment of patients to whom she is assigned.

Instruction in this phase of the curriculum, to have most meaning, must be patient-centered and family-centered if the student is to learn the full significance to the individual of being pregnant or of having a myocardial infarction, a stroke, a leg amputation, or a manic-depressive psychosis.

This third phase of the curriculum is primarily a series of experiences on the major clinical services of hospitals and other health agencies and in associated home care programs. In graduate curricula experience may be limited to the services of the student's choice or clinical specialty. The emphasis is on helping the patient to carry out his daily activities and the full range of diagnostic tests and treatments prescribed by the physician. In this phase the basic student must learn to function as she will be expected to function after she graduates. If in this phase she acquires independence in studying the patients she nurses, if she can learn about the patient through observing and listening to him, his family, and friends, if she can confer with other medical workers and use records and library resources effectively, she will possess the method by which she can, through the years, increase her nursing competence indefinitely.

It is essential that the student learn the value to the patient and the satisfaction to the nurse of this thorough type of patient study. Many basic students and some graduate nurses fail to experience what might be called "nursing in depth." In programs in which students are depended on for service they rarely have time for this individualized care. Nor can they envisage it if they never see graduate nurses practice it. Obviously, such nursing is dependent on a patient assignment system.

No attempt is made in this discussion to settle such a question as whether basic students should have experience in all divisions of the hospital, for example, the diet kitchens, the occupational and physical therapy departments, the outpatient departments, the operating and recovery rooms, and all units making up what we now call progressive patient care. The importance attached to the latter concept may result in a reorganization of hospitals so that students may be obliged to have experience in intensive- and self-care units, for example, in order to see patients in all stages of their illnesses. Nor can we go into the value of experience in nursery schools, nursing homes, or industrial health units.

Perhaps all I should stress is the importance of arranging the student's clinical, or field, experience so that it remains patient-centered. For example, I would advocate having students who are studying surgical nursing go with patients to the operating room, follow them into the recovery room, go back with them to the surgical unit, and finally follow them through clinics and home care services. This is in contrast to giving the student a month's experience in the operating suite, two weeks in the recovery room, a month in the outpatient department, and perhaps the same length of service in the home care program. If the emphasis is on the place rather than the patient, the teaching is likely to be focussed on how the unit operates, association with any one patient is limited, and the student cannot learn enough about him to give him much help.

Since we are accustomed to using blocks of experience in hospital departments as curriculum building units, it will be difficult to change the pattern. If, however, we are genuinely committed to the development of creative practitioners, we must make it possible for students to be with the patients to whom they are assigned over long periods of time and in different stages of their illnesses.

In Figure 11 the content suggested in the left-hand column might be presented as group instruction to the students on each of the services listed. Methods used will depend on the background of the instructors and students, the size of the groups, and the resources available. At this time, as in the second phase of the clinical curriculum, a panel of teachers can be very effective. For example, in discussing preparation for surgery the following persons can make distinct contributions: surgical and psychiatric nurses, a surgeon, an anesthetist, a social worker, a clergyman, and possibly a carefully chosen convalescent patient. In discussing prenatal care the nurse-midwife, the obstetrician, the social worker, the public health nurse, and the prospective parents are among those who can help the student develop a deep understanding of the satisfactions and anxieties of childbearing and the resources in the community for the promotion of maternal health and welfare.

The content suggested in the right-hand column of Figure 11 is most effectively taught, I believe, on a tutorial basis. That means helping the student, as she is assigned to a hydrocephalic infant, an alcoholic adult, or an acutely depressed suicidal adolescent, to study the nature of these conditions and their particular manifestations in the patients she is learning to help. If and when it is possible with benefit to the patient, clinics and conferences conducted around him may greatly enrich the student's understanding. Such sessions offer medical personnel a chance to pool their judgment. In most cases the patient and/or his family should be included but, in my opinion, the learning session fails if the patient or his relatives are frightened or embarrassed. Clinics and conferences are most successful when the participants are limited to those who know and serve the patient. When he senses that he is with friends who are trying to help him, he is usually able to discuss his problems, or his progress, with some degree of frankness. During such discussions students may acquire rare understanding of what it means, for example, to have tuberculosis, gout, diabetes, a drug addiction, or a spinal fracture.

The third phase of the clinical curriculum offers the student the opportunity to acquire the ability to find the related medical science that she needs. This is a rapidly developing field, and textbooks cannot be revised often enough to keep abreast of current therapy. Although instructors can help by providing bibliographies, students should be encouraged to use indexes, abstracts, and reviews and, in general, to develop habits of independent inquiry.

The ultimate measure of success in a curriculum based on the definition of nursing under discussion is the student's ability to help the patient with his daily regimen and to help him carry out the physician's therapeutic plan. In the first two phases of the curriculum she is functioning as a junior participant. In this last phase she must be able to perform the full range of nursing activities demanded by the needs of patients to whom she is assigned. She must also understand and be able to present orally and in writing the bases on which the diagnosis was made and the therapy prescribed. More especially she must be able to interpret to others her plan of nursing care and her reasons for following this particular plan.

If the student has learned the art of nursing, the individualization of care, and the ability to "get inside the patient's skin," she will be able to make a unique contribution to interdisciplinary patient conferences. Because she will be so closely identified with him, she may be, to some extent, the patient's voice when he is not a part of such conferences. The successful student will know something about the etiology of the patient's condition; she will have contributed to his rehabilitation throughout her care of him and will participate in making long-range plans to prevent recurrence of future dependence, if this is possible. Finally, with patients who cannot or did not recover she will have helped create conditions under which they could die in peace and with dignity.

Methods of Teaching

In discussing the kind of curriculum suggested by this concept of nursing, it has been impossible to avoid suggesting teaching methods—content and method are inseparable to some extent—so the following pages devoted to this topic may seem like a recapitulation; but, at the risk of being repetitious, I will again stress the value to the student of *observing* the expert practitioner, so much the better if she is a teacher-practitioner. In this event she will make it possible for the student to discuss the observation later. A reconstruction of the experience with a critical analysis will stimulate in the student an evaluative attitude toward patient-nurse interaction.

Observation as a first step in learning helps the student see the whole before she begins to study the parts. It is an antidote to the technical emphasis that is a result of crowding skills into the first nursing course. Job analyses have identified more than four hundred separate activities of nursing personnel. Granted that the effective generalist in nursing must ultimately master many procedures, it is a fatal mistake to overwhelm the student with them early in her program. The tendency in the past has been to teach in the first four months at least half the techniques the student will use throughout the entire practicum. If the criticism of nurses as technically expert but lacking in the more subtle arts of healing relationships is justified, this early lethal dose of technology may be an explanation.

I would suggest, therefore, that whenever a student is assigned to a new clinical service for practice (throughout the entire clinical curriculum) an experienced nurse work with her, allowing her at first to be a participant observer.

The student will feel awkward if she has nothing to do while she is observing, so it is, of course, desirable for her to acquire as soon as possible some of the basic skills that will enable her to work along with the experienced nurse whether the setting be a medical unit, a psychiatric service, or a home.

Giving the student this opportunity to observe and get her bearings has many advantages. As I have said, it shows her the whole before she is shown its parts. It gives her a chance to get interested in the patients whose care she observes. She identifies with them, and she sees the care through their eyes more than she would if she were responsible for it. Without this orientation period she is likely to be overwhelmed with all the new competences expected of her. As a result, her focus is on the impression she is creating, possibly on pleasing nurse administrators rather than on meeting the patient's needs.

To be of maximum benefit observation periods should be followed by analytical conferences or discussion periods. These may be informal, or they may be based on the student's written impressions or analysis of a tape-recorded observation period.

In teaching a specific skill there seems to be no substitute for a laboratory *demonstration*. The expert may demonstrate to one person or a roomful, depending upon the visibility. For this reason, and also because it is possible to stop it at any point, a demonstration on film is thought by some to have an advantage over a live one. It can also be perfected to an extent that is possible in few live demonstrations. On the other hand, the equipment and setting used in films may be different from those the student must practice with, and this is a disadvantage.

Because learning takes place, we believe, most readily when the learner is comfortable physically and emotionally, those watching a demonstration should be seated and, if possible, the subject should be exposed to no danger or physical harm, nor should he or she be embarrassed. For these reasons student nurses have been taught a wide range of skills on a manikin. But this has had the unfortunate effect of eliminating from the performance of nursing acts the interchange between nurse and patient that should accompany them. It also makes for unrealistic teaching.

If instructors are able and considerate, students will volunteer to be subjects for most laboratory demonstrations. In some cases the subject profits by experiencing the patient's role; in others she may be at a disadvantage because she can't see everything the demonstrator is doing.

Skills may be taught on a *tutoring* basis with the patient as the subject. The student in this case is a participant observer, and the patient need not sense that this is a learning session if he, the patient, remains the focus of the instructor's concern and if she is proficient in this sort of teaching. In my opinion the practice of bringing even a small group around a patient's bed for a demonstration is undesirable. The learners are physically uncomfortable and fear embarrassing the patient. The sensitive student who is most able to "get inside the patient's skin" (the potentially successful student) will be the most unhappy of the learners. This sacrifice of patient well-being to the learning needs of medical and nursing students is, I believe, a source of stress in their respective programs.

Regardless of the way in which a skill is demonstrated, *practice* should follow as soon as possible. Laboratories, or clinical classrooms, should be available and used throughout all phases of the nursing curriculum. Students gain greatly by practicing on each other. Except for the most readily learned or simple techniques, laboratory practice should precede clinical practice for the protection of both patient and student. Not until a student can inject a needle without acute anxiety should she be expected to give a hypodermic to a patient. (I remember a basic student who spent a half hour mustering up her courage to inject a hypodermic needle with the instructor acting as the subject.) Ideally the student who has practiced in the laboratory should first act as a graduate's assistant in carrying out the procedure with a patient. The next step is for the graduate to assist the student, and the last step is for the student to carry out the skill independently.

Individual conferences between students and instructors are used primarily to discuss patient problems and action the nursing staff might initiate in helping to solve them. It is in such teaching periods that the instructor and student review and evaluate what they have already done, trying to see where they succeeded and where they failed to help the patient. As suggested earlier, written reconstructions of patient-nurse interaction, or recorded incidents, help to make individual and group conferences effective.

Nursing clinics are sessions in which nurses and students assigned to the care of a particular patient meet to pool their knowledge about his situation and their judgment on how to help him. Usually the patient, a member of his family, or both, can, if they talk with this group, present a point of view that it is hard to introduce without them. However, some patients are too ill to participate; or for other reasons their participation may be contraindicated. Usually a graduate nurse or student presents the patient, which means reviewing his social and medical history briefly and giving, in much more detail, the difficulties his condition poses for him and the help that his nurses have been able to give. Particularly stressed are those problems for which a solution is sought and on which nursing judgment is to be pooled.

In one such clinic, to be specific, two tubercular patients recently transferred to a surgical unit worked through, with the nurses assigned to them, some of their dissatisfactions with their care, while the nurses were able to interpret some of the restrictions imposed on them because of the communicable nature of their illness. In another nursing clinic a daughter was helped, through discussion and demonstration, to plan for the terminal care of her father who wished to die at home. In the first case the patients were brought into the clinic session, in the second case a member of the family. In my opinion, basic as well as graduate nurse students should acquire the ability to plan and conduct such sessions.

In medical and some nursing schools similar clinical discussions are called "rounds." This comes from the practice of the instructing physician or nurse visiting each patient in turn ("making rounds") and teaching at the bedside a group of students that follow the instructor.

The desirability of this latter type of teaching is questionable. If the patient is on an open ward, his medical and social histories are reviewed in the hearing of fellow patients. This, I believe, is an invasion of his privacy. The students, too often, are not those assigned to him, so that the patient feels surrounded by strangers. Unless the instructor's remarks are directed to the patient, there is a tendency to use terminology that he does not understand. He may be frightened or embarrassed and misinterpret what is said by the medical personnel.

In my opinion, clinical teaching sessions focussed on the care of a patient should be held in a room designed for this purpose. Participants should be seated, and patients brought to the room for that part of the discussion to which they will contribute. Attention should be focussed on the patient, and any technical discussion that he might not be able to participate in or understand should be held before he joins the group or after he leaves it.

Interprofessional patient conferences can play an important part in clinical teaching programs for all health workers. Such a conference is a session in which the medical team serving the patient sits around a table, or in an informal group, and discusses the patient's condition, his needs, and what is being done or might be done to meet them. Patients and/or their families may come to the whole or a part of the conference. A physician, a nurse, a social worker, or any other professional worker might initiate the conference and act as chairman. Each type of worker contributes what he has learned by observation and by talking to the patient or to those who know him. At such a conference information on the nature of the disease, or condition, can be exchanged, and various therapeutic approaches or available health facilities discussed.

Any medical worker who is with the patient in a helping capacity may have something valuable to contribute to such a discussion. Certainly all who participate are in a better position to help the patient after the conference than they were before it.

In patient-centered interprofessional conferences, as in nursing or medical clinics, the discussion is more vital if the subject of it is present. In some cases he and/or his family may be asked to join in a part rather than the whole of the session. Obviously patient participation is likely to be better if the group is composed of workers he knows and who he believes are genuinely interested in his welfare.

In psychiatric hospitals this process of working through health problems in group discussion has been well developed.* It is, however, equally effective in other medical services. For example, during such a conference a forty-year-old woman scheduled to have an operation on her hands for deformities caused by gout was helped to realize that the conditions under which she lived were causing the acute attacks, or exacerbations, of the disease. From being completely dependent in the household of a married brother, she developed into a self-supporting individual who was able to make a home for herself and her mother. The nutritionist and physician who participated in this conference attributed the patient's increased self-understanding and the staff's increased helpfulness largely to the seeds planted in this group discussion.

* In 1930 I saw such conferences effectively used on the Psychiatric Service of the Strong Memorial Hospital in Rochester, New York. Dr. Eric Kent Clark was at that time the medical director of the unit and Miss Mary Maher the nurse director.

In another such interdisciplinary conference an elderly man with a recent amputation was helped to realize how many agencies there were in his community, such as sheltered workshops and recreational clubs for older people, that could help to keep his life reasonably normal in spite of his handicap. The staff as a whole was able to adopt a more hopeful and constructive approach to his care as a result of the many sources of help suggested.

Library research and study of community facilities are essential aspects of learning in the clinical curriculum. Reading is, in a sense, vicarious experience. If one could live forever, there might be an opportunity to learn firsthand all there is to know about the care of a depressed adult, a child with a cleft palate, or a young girl with pemphigus. But even if the learner might prefer this firsthand approach, the patient would suffer from his fumbling search for effective methods.

In order to have a safe minimum of knowledge about mankind in general and the individual's needs arising from his specific disease or condition, the nurse must extend her experience through reading. When she is given the opportunity to provide the full range of nursing care of the patient, and, most particularly, when she is conducting a nursing clinic or is acting as chairman of an interprofessional conference, she will need a thorough knowledge that can be acquired only through reading about all facets of the problems the patient presents and familiarizing herself with the community resources for helping the type of patient under consideration.

Children in the better grade schools and high schools of this country are given assignments that demand library research and investigation of community facilities. It cannot be assumed, however, that all high school graduates, or even college students, have competence along these lines. In any event, it is helpful to orient nursing students to the library resources to which they have access.

In discussing facilities I called attention to the importance of integrating hospital, medical, and nursing school libraries—

and even patient libraries. It is impossible in most situations to duplicate the holdings of journals, books and pamphlets, and most particularly the reference tools that all professional groups need. It is obviously more difficult to supply the service of librarians for two or three libraries than for one. Unstaffed or improperly staffed libraries are frustrating and soon develop in the users a distaste for the type of independent search of the literature that I believe nurses must make.

The nursing occupation has lagged in its efforts to produce guides to its literature. Some outstanding nursing periodicals lack indexes to their contents; few provide annual indexes and still fewer cumulative indexes. A current index to a limited number of periodicals has existed since 1956, and steps have been taken that will result in more extended periodical coverage in 1966.[80, 81, 82] The preparation of a sixty-year index to the analytical and historical aspects of the literature is in progress, and one volume is now available.[83]

Certain reference tools designed primarily for related medical and health personnel are useful to nurses. A few indexes, abstracts, excerpts, and bibliographies list publications on nursing or by nurses. The table on pages 100 to 110 shows types of reference tools.* It gives examples of those in related fields and lists the publications I believe available in each category that serve nursing primarily. In a library orientation for nursing students it is time well spent to show them all the tools designed for their occupation and the more important tools they must use in related fields, as for example those shown in the second column of this table.

* A study of this table shows the limitation of library tools in nursing and suggests a parallel limitation in library facilities. The largest national nursing library is, I believe, that of the Royal College of Nursing in London, England, with about 25,000 volumes. In this country there is no comparable unit, although the editorial library of the American Journal of Nursing Company, with about 5,000 volumes, has served in this capacity. Although the National Library of Medicine and some large university libraries (with one or more *million* volumes) may have relatively good nursing collections, the profession needs national and regional centers where scholars can depend upon finding all significant publications on nursing.

As I have implied, *audiovisual* aids can and should be used freely in connection with the clinical nursing program. It is always more effective to show an object or a process than merely to talk about it. There are hundreds of films with sound tracks, film strips, and slides that supplement the opportunities for learning within the school and related field agencies. A school lacking projection equipment is seriously handicapped, as is the instructor who cannot operate it.

Recordings of nurse-patient interaction and even lectures may be used as a basis for group discussion. The former, if accompanied by commentaries or evaluations, might be kept where the student could listen to them as she might read books.

Experiments with *television* suggest that it may be used to extend teaching personnel not only in demonstrating (as we've suggested earlier) but also in helping students with practice or experience on clinical services. With a system of closed-circuit television, one instructor at a monitor's station can be available to students in a number of wards or rooms simultaneously.

Having had no firsthand experience with this use of television, I am unprepared to make specific recommendations, except to suggest that it warrants continued investigation. It certainly can be used in evaluating student performance and in some kinds of clinical research. Each student is provided with a mechanism that enables her to talk with the instructor. Current experiments suggest that such communication between the teacher and learner is not altogether satisfactory; rather that the student hesitates to ask questions in the patient's hearing.[84, 85, 86, 87, 88]

Programmed instruction, with and without *teaching machines,* is discussed in the literature. Not having used this method, I, again, hesitate to suggest anything more than that the reader study it and that the nursing occupation continue to experiment with it. Programmed instruction is designed primarily for units of content that the student can learn without the presence of the instructor if he is adequately guided by printed instructions and audiovisual aids. It is carefully planned to test the student's understanding of each step before he goes on to the next—and this is where the machine is particularly helpful. With the machine, the student cannot proceed until he gives the right answer. The particular merits of this procedure are that the student has immediate satisfaction from success, or knows when he is succeeding, and can progress at his or her own speed. Properly used, it should conserve the instructor's time so that he is available when his presence is most needed.[89, 90, 91]

Group and individual projects that involve student presentations are useful in developing ability to share knowledge and skills. One of the functions of the nurse is to teach patients or members of their families. She is expected to give general health guidance and to help others to acquire competence in procedures such as giving hypodermic injections, operating inhalation equipment or even, most recently, the units that perform the function of the kidney when there is permanent kidney damage. She may be a leader in child care discussion, or she may conduct a session in group therapy.

It is obvious that experience with peer groups will help the student learn to feel comfortable in the teaching, or guiding, role. Obviously her field experience must give her an opportunity to see expert nurses teaching individual patients before she is expected to do so.

Actually almost every teaching method I know is suited to some part of the clinical program if the teacher uses it judiciously. *Lectures* are not stressed because they have been so overused and misused in the past. Nurse instructors and physicians have talked about patients, equipment, skills, and therapies that they could have shown. I, for instance, have listened to an elaborate lecture on a respirator with only mention made of the fact that the machine itself could be seen in such and such a room. Nor was there any indication that the lecture would be followed by a demonstration. This is a case in which a demonstration was indicated. This should have been followed by practice, with the students acting as subjects, then by participant observation, and finally full participation with independent care of patients in respirators. Any lecture given should have been in conjunction with a demonstration of the machine and its operation.

In my opinion lectures are most effectively used to introduce a broad topic as, for example, the function of the nurse, planning nursing care, providing for continuity of care, the problem of long-term illness, or the posthospital care of the psychiatric patient. It may also be the best method to use in rounding out any one of such topics.

Recitations based on textbooks are mentioned in this discussion only to relegate them to what I hope is a dead era. In the past students were assigned a chapter of a text. The instructor, with the text before her, questioned students to see how much they remembered of what they had, supposedly, read. The result was that poor students were embarrassed and the scholar's time was wasted. There are other means, such as written tests and discussions in which sources are cited, that make the students feel responsible for a common body of knowledge represented by texts and other assigned readings.

Evaluation of student progress has had so much attention in the literature that the inquiring faculty finds ample help. This does not mean that we know all we want to know about testing and measuring. But studies show that there is a close relationship between accomplishment on written tests and clinical ability of students as judged by those who work with them. For this reason we have relied heavily on written tests. In this country, at least, comprehensive examinations have been developed for which national low, average, and superior accomplishments are known. Because preparatory schools differ regionally, some educators think we should not use national standards. In my opinion, we can use these nationally developed tests and at the same time make those adjustments and modifications demanded by the particular program concerned.

Although we may rely on written tests for grades, very largely, the emphasis in evaluation as a teaching tool should be based on how effectively the student helps patients to carry out their daily regimens and utilize therapeutic resources. The ultimate aim of evaluation is to make the student self-critical or to recognize her successes and her failures and the reasons for them. If the instructor has a helping rather than a judgmental relationship with the student, the latter can develop this analytical attitude toward her work. She is not always pretending that she knows what she thinks she is supposed to know or able to carry out treatments about which she is very insecure.

Summary

To some readers the foregoing suggestions on nursing education may offer little that is new; to others they imply a complete revamping of the curriculum. The first group may not be especially interested; the latter may be discouraged.

Perhaps we should all recognize that revision of established patterns of nursing education calls for strong leadership, that it is not easy to accomplish.

Since the turn of the century prominent American nurses and physicians here and abroad have said that nursing programs should be developed within the educational system of the country concerned rather than within service agencies, where most of them still are. Miss Nutting and Miss Goodrich are two who spoke most cogently for nursing; Dr. Welch, Dr. Beard, and Dr. Lyons for medicine.[92, 93, 94, 95, 96] In 1954 Dr. Robson of the University of Adelaide in Australia wrote on "the need for a revolution in the nursing profession." He said, "Educational methods are failing to keep pace with the needs. . . . the present system as it stands today in Australia, and in many other countries, is archaic and inadequate. . . . I would suggest unhesitatingly that the educational program should be raised to university standards."[97]

Another Australian physician, John Lindell, writing on nursing as a profession, said, "Nurse training has not kept pace with medical progress though doctors often assume that it has." He went on to say that the duties of the nurse ". . . embrace the whole field of patient care from the simplest menial task to work involving a sound knowledge of physics, chemistry, physiology, and bacteriology." Later he referred to the nurse as a "professional colleague" of the doctor.[98] Dr. Crew, commenting on the English system, said, "The cost of training has never been adequately faced. . . ." Speaking of the inadequacy even of the endowed Nightingale School at St. Thomas's, he said, "The constant stream of eager recruits to nursing was far too profitable to the hospital and no one had the vision to suggest that nursing should come within the educational system of the country."[99] Dr. René Sand, the Belgian physician and international health expert, referring to the nurse as the "sentinel of health," attributed to her influence alone the 42 per cent reduction in deaths from measles and 89 per cent in scarlet fever between 1920 and 1935 for, he said, the doctors introduced no new methods of treating or preventing children's illnesses in this period. He spoke of her work as "unending" and said her knowledge was to be "all embracing."[100]

Dr. H. E. MacDermot, writing on "Nursing in Osler's Student Days," conjectured that he must have been influenced by the attitude of Dr. R. P. Howard, one of his teachers. He said that Dr. Howard advocated a liberal education for the nurse similar to that of the doctor with a three-year professional education following, and he thought that nursing should be elevated to a scientific art.[101]

Many of us believe that medical care will never reach its fullest development until a peer relationship is established among those in the health professions. In order to accomplish optimum cooperation, these professions must speak a common language (this does not mean jargon). A common background for the students is one means of achieving this mutual understanding, and a common core of professional knowledge is another. Prospective students of medicine, nursing, social work, and clinical psychology would profit, for example, by studying the same physical, biological, and social sciences. Later, in their respective professional programs, a core content could be identified that they would study together. Having known each other and worked together in undergraduate and graduate courses, they would find it a natural process as practitioners to confer on patient care. The final test of each health worker is how effectively he or she can work with other health and welfare workers in the community who serve the patient and his family.

At a meeting twenty years ago when someone was bemoaning the fact that there were no leaders in nursing coming along to take the place of our great women of the past, Miss Goodrich rose to protest. She said the conditions are passing that demand the militant personalities of earlier years. She maintained that the *idea* should lead—not the individual. She believed that all of us in the fields of health and welfare have a common goal— the improved lot of the individual. She assumed that the definition of health in the World Health Organization's charter (a state of complete physical, mental, and social well-being, and not merely the absence of disease or infirmity) is indeed our goal. I think she believed, as I do, that the doctor, the nurse, the social worker, the nutritionist, the physical therapist, the occupational consultant, and others must work together as true partners in this effort to help the individual realize his potential. She saw as inevitable, rather than as something nurses must fight for, the preparation of all these workers within the colleges and universities. She believed, beyond the shadow of a doubt, that what she called "the complete nurse"—the woman with social experience and a thorough education—had proved her worth, not only as administrator and teacher but more particularly as a practitioner.*

I think that the professional quality of nursing service and the appropriateness of a professional preparation has been

* The struggle to make nursing education comparable to that of other occupations giving a complex service to mankind is a long and hard one. Charles H. Russell's survey of the literature on a liberal education for the nurse is pertinent, and those interested in this subject will find it rewarding. (Russell, Charles H.: Liberal Education and Nursing. *Nurs. Res.*, 7:116–26, [Fall] 1958).

grasped in many countries, but that the means by which these
ideas can be implemented are slow in developing. It is up to us
who share this faith in the social value of nursing to speed this
process.

Miss L. M. Avery, an Australian nurse, makes an observation
worth thinking about. She said, "To me nursing is like a seed
planted in very arid soil, which by nourishment, constant loving
care and attention, grew into a sturdy tree with promise of future growth. We have been content to sit in the shade of its
branches, forgetting that it is still a young tree requiring constant supervision and nourishment."[102]

In final summary, I believe that the function the nurse
performs is primarily an independent one—that of acting for the
patient when he lacks knowledge, physical strength, or the will
to act for himself as he would ordinarily act in health, or in
carrying out prescribed therapy. This function is seen as complex and creative, as offering unlimited opportunity for the application of the physical, biological, and social sciences, and the
development of skills based on them. I believe society wants
and expects this service from the nurse and that no other worker
is as able, or willing, to give it.

If a nurse believes that she is pre-eminent in an area of
health practice, she will try to develop a working milieu in
which she can realize her potential value to the person served.
She will also recognize her responsibility for the validation and
improvement of methods she uses—or her responsibility for
clinical nursing research.

In order to practice as an expert in her own right and to
use the scientific approach to the improvement of practice, the
nurse needs the kind of education that, in our society, is available only in colleges and universities. Training programs operated on funds pinched from the budgets of service agencies
cannot provide the preparation the nurse needs. Her work demands a universal sympathy for, and understanding of, diverse
human beings. The liberalizing effect of a general education

must be recognized since the personality of the nurse is possibly the most important intangible in measuring the effect of nursing care. I can think of no better ending than to cite Claire Dennison's conclusion that "Finally and fundamentally the quality of nursing care depends upon the quality of those giving care."[103]

ADDENDUM
IMPLICATIONS FOR NURSING EDUCATION

There is nothing that dominates this era more than the extent and rapidity of change. Stephen Hawking, the scientist now on the faculty of Cambridge University who writes for the public under the all-embracing title *A Brief History of Time,* shows this rapidity of change by discussing the hundreds of scientific discoveries—in thought and practice—in this age that parallel a dozen or so scientific principles that have dominated the science of past ages. Luther Christman, former dean and nurse administrator at Rush University in Chicago, writes today about many scientific principles of recent origin that affect nursing administration, principles that if known and applied would materially affect the practice of nurse administrators.

This application of general principles should be part of any effort to improve or advance a profession. In nursing education today, the idea that students adopt the "theory" of another person and practice according to this theory is, I believe, an unfortunate viewpoint. I would stress, writing today, that students study existing theories but realize that the guiding concept should be one's own. The amalgam of the many concepts they study may be different from any other—it may be unique just as every person is unique.

The modification in my concept of nursing since I wrote *The Nature of Nursing* in 1966 suggests a different emphasis, at least, on nursing education. I recognize now, as I think the majority of health care providers recognize, that registered nurses or their equivalents are the major providers of primary care. Obstetrical nurses, or midwives, have been universally recognized worldwide as the providers of primary care for mothers and newborns. They diagnose and treat as well as "care" for mothers and infants; midwives are educated to diagnose, to treat, as well as to care.

This question of the extent or range of the nurse's function is affected in every society by the numbers of providers of diagnosis, treatment, and care available. Where therapists predominate, as in India, for example, the functions of doctors and nurses differ from those in the United States where nurses are the overwhelming majority.

Since nurses and midwives in the United States do diagnose and treat, as well as care for their clients or patients, their educational preparation should include appropriate evaluation, knowledge, and skills. If I were writing this book today, I would emphasize the importance of preparing all nurses for this wider range of functions than was emphasized in 1966. Such preparation should apply to *continuing* education also, because methods of diagnosis and treatment are never static.

LIBRARY TOOLS FOR NURSING

(Those published in English and available in the United States)

Types	Examples of References for Health Fields Which, in Some Cases, Include Nursing	References Prepared for the Field of Nursing
ABSTRACTS AND EXCERPTS	*Dissertation Abstracts.* Abstracts of Dissertations and Monographs in Microfilm, Ann Arbor, Mich., University Microfilms, Inc. Published monthly with annual compilations since 1940. Includes publications on nursing, nursing education, and nurses. *Hospital Abstracts.* Printed and distributed by H. M. Stationery Office, London. Monthly survey of world literature since 1961. Prepared by Great Britain's Ministry of Health. Includes entries on hospital nursing and nurses. *Psychological Abstracts.* American Psychological Association, Washington. Published monthly with annual compilations since 1940. Represents search of more than 400 journals, some of which carry articles on nursing and nurses.	"Abstracts of Studies in Public Health Nursing 1924–1957." In *Nursing Research* **8**:45–115, Spring, 1959. Prepared under the direction of Hortense Hilbert, Institute of Research and Service in Nursing Education, Teachers College, Columbia University, New York. Represents search of many monographic listings and articles selected from 21 periodicals. "Abstracts of Reports of Studies in Nursing." In *Nursing Research* since 1960. Regular department of this journal now prepared under the direction of the American Nurses Foundation, New York. Represents search of many monographic listings and more than 200 periodicals.
BIBLIOGRAPHIES	*Bibliography of Reproduction.* A classified title list compiled from the world's literature. Reproduction Research Information Service, Cambridge, Eng. Monthly publication with annual compilation since 1963. *Bibliography of Medical Reviews.* Prepared under the direction of the Bibliographic Services Division, National Library of Medicine, Washington. Printed and distributed by U.S. Government Printing Office, Washington.	*A Bio-Bibliography of Florence Nightingale.* Prepared by William J. Bishop and Sue Goldie for the International Council of Nurses with which is associated the Florence Nightingale Foundation, London. Printed by Dawsons of Pall Mall, London, England, 1962, 162 p. (Nursing schools as, for example, those at the Columbia-Presbyterian Medical Center, New York, and the University of Kansas, Kansas City, Kan., have also

Types	Examples of References for Health Fields Which, in Some Cases, Include Nursing	References Prepared for the Field of Nursing
BIBLIOGRAPHIES *(continued)*	Published monthly with annual compilations since 1956.	published catalogues of their collections of Nightingalia.)

Bibliography of Medical Translations, Jan. 1959–June 1962. Prepared by the Office of Technical Services, U.S. Department of Commerce, Washington. Printed and distributed by U.S. Government Printing Office, Washington, 1963, various pagings.

Medical Behavioral Science. A selected bibliography of cultural anthropology, social psychology, and sociology in medicine. Prepared by Marion Pearsall. Published and distributed by University of Kentucky Press, Lexington, 1963, 134 p.

Poliomyelitis Current Literature: A Periodical Annotated List. Issued monthly from 1945 to 1962 by the Library of the National Foundation for Infantile Paralysis, New York. Classified author and subject list.

Bibliographies on Nursing. Prepared by committees of its members for the National League for Nursing, New York. Published and distributed by the League, 1957, 14 vols. (Out of print.) Books, pamphlets, periodical articles, films, and other audiovisual aids briefly described and arranged in 32 subject listings.

Bibliography on Cancer for Nurses, Annotated. Prepared by Patricia B. Geiser, U.S. Public Health Service, Washington. Printed and distributed by U.S. Government Printing Office, Washington, 1959, 38 p. Classified list of books, pamphlets, and periodical articles.

Basic Book and Periodical List for Nursing School and Medical Library. 3 ed., 1961, 100 p. *Supplement to Basic Book . . . 1963,* 52 p. *Source Book of Free and Low Cost Materials for Medical and Nursing School Libraries, 1961,* 33 p. Prepared by Sister M. Concordia, Library of the Queen of Angels School of Nursing, Los Angeles. Distributed by the Library.

Reference Tools for Nursing. Prepared by the Interagency Council for Library Tools for Nursing, 1964, 9 p. Distributed by the Library of the American Journal of Nursing Co., New York. Selected classified list of books, pamphlets, and periodical publications.

Types	Examples of References for Health Fields Which, in Some Cases, Include Nursing	References Prepared for the Field of Nursing
CATALOGUES	*National Library of Medicine Catalogue.* Part I, Authors; Part II, Subjects. Prepared jointly by Library of Congress and National Library of Medicine, Washington. This publication represents the latter's card catalogue. With the *Index Medicus* it is the published monthly record of the monographic and periodical holdings of the National Library of Medicine. Annual Compilation for 1963, 6 vols. Published and distributed by the Library, Washington.	*The Adelaide Nutting Historical Nursing Collection, Teachers College, Columbia University, New York City.* Prepared under the direction of Isabel M. Stewart, Department of Nursing Education. Published and distributed by Bureau of Publications, Teachers College, 1929, 68 p. Classified list of books, pamphlets, letters, journal and newspaper articles.
	National Union Catalogue. Prepared by National Library of Congress with cooperation of Committee on Resources of American Libraries, American Library Association, Chicago. Monthly listing by author of Library of Congress cards and titles reported to other American libraries. Compilation for 1958–1962 published by Rowman and Littlefied, New York, 54 vols. (Includes motion picture and filmstrip titles.)	
DICTIONARIES (AND A THESAURUS)	*Dictionary of the Social Sciences.* Edited by Julius Gould and William L. Kolb. Compiled under the auspices of United Nations Educational Scientific and Cultural Organization, Paris and New York. Published and distributed by the Free Press of Glencoe, a Division of The Macmillan Co., New York, 1964, 761 p. Contributions from many countries describe and define	*American Nurses Dictionary.* Prepared by Alice Louise Price. Published and distributed by W. B. Saunders Co., Philadelphia, 1949, 656 p. Alphabetical list of definitions and pronunciations of terms used by nurses.

Types	Examples of References for Health Fields Which, in Some Cases, Include Nursing	References Prepared for the Field of Nursing
DICTIONARIES (AND A THESAURUS) *(continued)*	about 1000 concepts. Arranged alphabetically. *Medical and Health Sciences Thesaurus.* Prepared under the direction of Dale R. Lindsay, National Institutes of Health, Bethesda, Md. Printed and distributed by U.S. Government Printing Office, Washington, D.C., 1963, 212 p. Alphabetical list of related terms. *The Origin of Medical Terms,* 2 ed. Prepared by Henry Alan Skinner. Published and distributed by William & Wilkins Co., Baltimore, 1961, 437 p. Alphabetical list with biographical notes and drawings of many physicians involved. *Psychiatric Dictionary,* 3 ed. Prepared by Leland E. Hinsie and R. J. Campbell. Published and distributed by Oxford Press, New York, 1960, 788 p. *Standard Nomenclature of Disease and Operations,* 5 ed. Edited by Edward T. Thompson and Adeline C. Hayden. Published and distributed by Blakiston, McGraw-Hill Book Co., New York, 1961, 964 p.	
DIRECTORIES (PERSONS, AGENCIES, INSTITUTIONS, ORGANIZA- TIONS)	*American Medical Directory—A Register of Physicians,* 22 ed. Prepared, published, and distributed by The American Medical Association, Chicago, 1963, 1824 p. *American Public Health Association Membership Directory.*	*Educational Programs in Nursing.* Prepared, published, and distributed by National League for Nursing, New York. Annual classified list. *Catholic Education Programs for Nurses.* Prepared by Catholic Hospital Association;

Types	Examples of References for Health Fields Which, in Some Cases, Include Nursing	References Prepared for the Field of Nursing
DIRECTORIES (PERSONS, AGENCIES, INSTITUTIONS, ORGANIZA-TIONS) *(continued)*	Prepared, published, and distributed by the Association, New York, 1962, 408 p. *Foundation Directory,* 2 ed. Prepared, published, and distributed by The Foundation Library Center, Russell Sage Foundation, New York, 1964, 1000 p. *Mental Health Directory of State and National Agencies Administering Public Mental Health and Related Programs, 1964.* Prepared under the direction of R. H. Felix, National Institutes of Health, Bethesda, Md. Printed and distributed by U.S. Government Printing Office, Washington, D.C., 1964, 156 p. *Scientific and Technical Societies of The United States and Canada,* 7 ed. Prepared under the direction of John H. Gribbin, National Academy of Sciences, National Research Council, Washington. Published and distributed by the Council, 1961. Part I, *The United States,* 413 p. Part II, *Canada,* 54 p. Alphabetical list, giving history, purpose, membership, and other date on societies. *Study Abroad; International Directory of Fellowships, Scholarships, and Awards, 1964–1966,* 15 ed. Compiled by United Nations Educational, Scientific, and Cultural Organization. Published and distributed The UNESCO Publications Center, Paris, Fr. and New York, 1963, 643 p. Includes list by sponsoring organizations and by countries, arranged alphabetically. Information in English, French, and Spanish.	published annually by the American Hospital Association in its journal *Hospitals.* *Official Directory of International, National and State Nursing Organizations [and Some Related Organizations].* Prepared and published semi-annually by the American Journal of Nursing Company in its periodicals, *The American Journal of Nursing* and *Nursing Outlook* State Registered Nurses. Lists prepared in each state by its board of registry. Restricted lists, not generally available. State Nurses' Associations' Memberships. Lists prepared by headquarters staffs of State Nurses' Associations. Restricted lists, not generally available.

Types	Examples of References for Health Fields Which, in Some Cases, Include Nursing	References Prepared for the Field of Nursing
ENCYCLOPEDIAS	*Encyclopedia of Associations.* Vol. I, *National Organizations of the United States.* Vol. II, *Geographic-Executive Index.* Edited by Frederick C. Ruffner, *et al.* Published and distributed by Gale Research Co., Detroit, 1964. Classified list. *Encyclopedia of Medical Syndromes.* Prepared by Robert H. Durham. New York, Paul B. Hoeber, Inc. (Medical Division of Harpers) 1960, 628 p. *Encyclopedia of Social Work* (Successor to *Social Work Year Book*). Edited by Harry L. Lurie for National Association of Social Workers, New York. Published and distributed by the Association, 1965, 1060 p. Includes articles, biography, statistics, directory of agencies, list of periodicals, code of ethics, and definition of social work.	*The Encyclopedia of Nursing.* Prepared under the supervision of Lucile Petry. Published and distributed by W. B. Saunders, Philadelphia, 1952, 1009 p. Alphabetical list. Coverage based on analysis of terms used in nursing texts.
HANDBOOKS OR MANUALS	*Handbook of Medical Library Practice,* 2 ed. Edited by Janet Doe and Mary L. Marshall for the American Medical Library Association, Chicago, 1956, 601 p. Includes 1,965 references of which 20 are on nursing. Published and distributed by the Association. *Handbook of Social Psychology.* Vol. I, *Theory and Method.* Vol. II, *Special Fields and Applications.* Prepared by Gardner Lindzey, Harvard University, Cambridge, Mass. Published and distributed by Addison-Wesley Publishing Co., Reading [Mass.]	*Library Handbook for Schools of Nursing,* 2 ed. Revision by Committee of the National League of Nursing Education, New York, Deborah M. Jensen, Chairman. Published and distributed by National League for Nursing, New York, 1953, 265 p. Makes recommendations on organizing and administering a library's building and equipping it. Lists subject headings and classification for contents, or entries. *Lippincott's Quick Reference Book for Nurses,* 7 ed. Prepared by Helen Young, *et al.*

Types	Examples of References for Health Fields Which, in Some Cases, Include Nursing	References Prepared for the Field of Nursing
HANDBOOKS OR MANUALS *(continued)*	and London, Eng., 1954. 2 vols. Compilation of articles by many contributors who review the literature and append bibliographies. *New and Nonofficial Drugs.* Prepared under the direction of John R. Lewis for the Council on Drugs of the American Medical Association, Chicago. Annually since 1913. Now published by J. B. Lippincott Co., Philadelphia. Alphabetical list of drugs with information on each. *United States Government Organization Manual, 1964–1965.* Prepared under the direction of Wayne C. Grover, National Archives and Records Service, General Services Administration, Washington. Printed and distributed by U.S. Government Printing Office, Washington, D.C., 1964, 784 p. Gives brief history of departments and agencies and their dependent divisions and bureaus. Some diagrams showing relationships.	Published and distributed by J. B. Lippincott Co., Philadelphia, 1955, 727 p. Compilation of information related chiefly to hospital nursing practice.
INDEXES	*Cancer Current Literature Index.* Prepared by Excerpta Medica Foundation, New York, and Amsterdam, Neth. Published and distributed by American Cancer Society, Inc., New York. Since 1959 (irregular). *A Cumulative Index to a Continuing Bibliography on Aerospace Medicine and Biology.* Prepared by the National Aeronautics and Space Administration, Washington, 1965, various pagings. Subject and author listing.	*American Journal of Nursing; Annual and Cumulative Indexes.* These and Reference Card Service prepared under direction of Lois B. Miller for American Journal of Nursing Co., New York, 1900–. Combined subject and author listing. *Cumulative Index to Nursing Literature.* Prepared under the direction of Mildred Grandbois, *et al.* Glendale Sanitarium and Hospital Publication Service, Glendale, Calif. Now

Types	Examples of References for Health Fields Which, in Some Cases, Include Nursing	References Prepared for the Field of Nursing
INDEXES (continued)	*Hospital Literature Index.* Prepared by the Library Staff of the American Hospital Association, Chicago. Published and distributed by the Association since 1945. Quarterly (with annual compilations). Subject-author index of books and pamphlets and articles from more than 300 periodicals, including 16 nursing journals. *Index Medicus.* Prepared by the National Library of Medicine, Washington, since 1960. Printed and distributed by U.S. Government Printing Office. Monthly, with annual compilations. Author and subject guide to more than 5000 journals. Current list includes 7 nursing journals. Supplants index with same title published by American Medical Association and *Current List of Medical Literature,* published by the National Library of Medicine. *International Index; Quarterly Guide to Periodical Literature in the Social Sciences and Humanities.* Prepared and published by the H. W. Wilson Co., New York. Subject and author listing. *Psychiatric Index for Interdisciplinary Research: A Guide to the Literature, 1950–1961.* Edited by Richard A. Schermerhorn, Western Reserve University. Prepared under the auspices of U.S. Vocational Rehabilitation Administration, Washington. Printed and distrib-	published quarterly, with annual compilations, since 1956. Subject and author guide to 54 periodicals in nursing and related fields. *International Nursing Index to Periodical Literature.* Announced for publication in 1966 by The American Journal of Nursing Company, New York, in collaboration with the National Library of Medicine, Bethesda, Md. *Nursing Outlook; Annual and Cumulative Indexes.* These and Reference Card Service prepared under the direction of Lois B. Miller for the American Journal of Nursing Co., New York, 1953–. Combined subject and author listing. *Nursing Research; Annual and Cumulative Indexes.* These and Reference Card Service prepared under the direction of Lois B. Miller for the American Journal of Nursing Co., New York, 1952–. Combined subject and author listing. *Nursing Studies Index: An Annotated Guide to Reported Studies, Research in Progress, Research Methods and Historical Materials in Periodicals, Books and Pamphlets Published in English.* Prepared under the direction of Virginia Henderson by the Yale University School of Nursing Index Staff, New Haven, Conn. Published and distributed by J. B.

Types	Examples of References for Health Fields Which, in Some Cases, Include Nursing	References Prepared for the Field of Nursing
INDEXES *(continued)*	uted by U.S. Government Printing Office, Washington, 1964, 1249 p. Alphabetical author list of articles, under 71 categories, selected from 124 periodicals, including 1 nursing journal. *Research Grants Index: Fiscal Year 1963.* Vol. I, *Index Section.* Vol. II, *Grant Number List and Bibliography, General Research Areas, and Alphabetical Listing of Investigators.* Third edition of this index prepared under direction of Eugene A. Confrey and Lynda Cahoon McGee, Division of Research Grants, National Institutes of Health, U.S. Public Health Service, Bethesda, Md. Printed and distributed by U.S. Government Printing Office, Washington, 1964, 2 vols.	Lippincott Co., Philadelphia. Vol. IV (1957–1959), 1963, 281 p. Vol. III (1950–1956) in publication. Vols. II (1930–1949) and I (1900–1929), in preparation. Alphabetical subject and author lists of books and pamphlets and of articles selected from more than 200 periodicals searched.
INVENTORIES AND LISTS	*Inventory of Social and Economic Research in Health.* Prepared, published, and distributed by the Health Information Foundation, New York, since 1952. Annual classified list of current research, giving staff, sponsorship, source of support, and method of investigation. Many studies involve nursing or nurses. *New Serial Titles. A Union List of Serials Commencing Publication After Dec. 31, 1949.* Prepared, published, and distributed by U.S. Library of Congress, Washington, 1963, 2035 p.	*Clearing House List of Studies in Nursing, 1950–1955.* Supplements, 1955–1956, 1957–1958, and 1959–1961. Prepared under the direction of Clara A. Hardin, Research and Statistics Unit, American Nurses Association, New York. Published and distributed by the Association. Classified list. *List of Advanced Programs in Nursing Education (1951–52) and Supplement to List . . . (1957).* Prepared by the Florence Nightingale Foundation, which is associated with the International Council of Nurses, London, Eng., 1958.

Types	Examples of References for Health Fields Which, in Some Cases, Include Nursing	References Prepared for the Field of Nursing
INVENTORIES AND LISTS *(continued)*	*Union List of Serials in Libraries of The United States and Canada,* 2 ed. Edited by Mary Frank, *et al.* Published and distributed by H. W. Wilson Co., New York, 1953, 1365 p.	Number, type, and duration of programs described and shown diagrammatically. *The Nation's Nurses: The 1962 Inventory of Professional Registered Nurses.* Prepared by Elinor D. Marshall and Evelyn B. Moses, Research and Statistics Program, American Nurses Association, New York. Published and distributed by the Association, 1965, 34 p. Compilation of data on characteristics of the nurse supply and educational preparation of nurses in areas of clinical practice in selected states. Supplants data assembled in 1956–1958 inventory.
REVIEWS, SURVEYS, AND SOURCE BOOKS	*Excerpta Medica [A World Guide].* Excerpta Medica Foundation, New York and Amsterdam, Neth. Published monthly (with annual compilations) through international cooperation of specialists, in 19 sections according to medical specialities as, for example, Internal Medicine, Chest Diseases, and Pediatrics. *Review of Child Development Research.* Prepared by Martin L. Hoffman and Lois Wladis Hoffman. Published and distributed by Russell Sage Foundation, 1964, 547 p. *Sociological Studies of Health and Sickness: A Source Book for the Health Professions.* Prepared by Dorian Apple. Published and distributed by	*History of Nursing Source Book.* Prepared by Anne L. Austin. Published and distributed by G. P. Putnam's Sons, New York, 1957, 480 p. Excerpts from writings on nursing and nurses from Biblical times. *Nursing Research; A Survey and Assessment.* Prepared by Leo W. Simmons and Virginia Henderson. Published and distributed by Appleton-Century-Crofts, New York, 1964, 461 p. Discusses development of research and major studies in selected areas. Includes classification scheme, bibliography, and list of doctoral dissertations by nurses.

Types	Examples of References for Health Fields Which, in Some Cases, Include Nursing	References Prepared for the Field of Nursing
REVIEWS, SURVEYS, AND SOURCE BOOKS *(continued)*	McGraw-Hill Book Co., New York, 1960, 350 p. Annotated classified guide that includes studies on nursing and nurses.	
STATISTICAL GUIDES	*Statistical Abstract of the United States, 1963,* 84 ed. Prepared under the direction of Edwin A. Goldfield, U.S. Department of Commerce, Washington. Published and distributed by U.S. Government Printing Office, 1963, 1036 p. Annual compilation. Includes data on nurses, hospitals, nursing homes, patients, and a wide variety of subjects of interest to the nursing occupation. *Statistics Sources.* Edited by Paul Wasserman, *et al.* Published and distributed by Gale Research Co., Detroit, 1962, 288 p. Alphabetical guide to current sources of statistical data.	*Facts About Nursing.* Prepared under the direction of Elinor D. Marshall, Research and Statistics Program, American Nurses Association, New York. Published and distributed by the Association since 1935. 1962–1963 ed., 256 p. Annual compendium that includes data on numbers and distribution of nurses, employment conditions, numbers of students, graduations, withdrawals, and types of programs. Also contains a directory of major international and national nursing organizations and statements on their purposes.
YEARBOOKS	*Occupational Therapy Yearbook, 1961.* Prepared, published, and distributed by the Occupational Therapy Association, New York, 1961, 360 p. Contains directory of members, list of hospitals having occupational therapy departments, educational standards, and the Constitution of the Association. *The Practical Medicine Yearbook.* Prepared, published, and distributed by Year Book Medical Publishers, Chicago, since 1900. Series for 1964–1965 in 17 vols. A large editorial staff attempts to give, in abstract form, the essence of international medico-scientific literature.	*The Yearbook of Modern Nursing.* Edited by M. Cordelia Cowan. Published and distributed by G. P. Putnam's Sons, New York, 1956, 1957–1958, and 1959. Many contributors review the literature on organizations in nursing, trends, nursing education, research, and practice in major clinical fields.

References

1. Nightingale, Florence: *Notes on Nursing. What It Is and What It Is Not* (facsimile of 1859 ed.). J. B. Lippincott Co., Philadelphia, 1946, p. 79.
2. Taylor, Effie J.: Of What Is the Nature of Nursing? *Amer. J. Nurs.,* **34:**476, (May) 1934.
3. _____: A Concept of Nursing. *Amer. J. Nurs.,* **33:**565, (June) 1933.
4. Goodrich, Annie W.: *A Definition of Nursing.* Privately printed leaflet, 1946, p. 2.
5. Report of the Biennial. *Amer. J. Nurs.,* **47:**471, (Nov.) 1946.
6. Brown, Esther Lucile: *Nursing for the Future.* Russell Sage Foundation, New York, 1948, p. 198.
7. National Nursing Council, Inc.: *A Thousand Think Together. A Report of Three Regional Conferences Held in Connection with the Study of Schools of Nursing.* New York, The Council, 1948, lv. 209.
8. Hughes, Everett C., et al.: *Twenty Thousand Nurses Tell Their Story.* J. B. Lippincott Co., Philadelphia, 1958, p. 280.
9. ANA Statement. Auxiliary Personnel in Nursing Service. *Amer. J. Nurs.,* **62:**72, (July) 1962.
10. ANA Board Approves a Definition of Nursing Practice. *Amer. J. Nurs.,* **55:**1474, (Dec.) 1955.
11. Professional Nursing Defined. *Amer. J. Nurs.,* **37:**578, (May) 1937.
12. Hershey, Nathan: The Law and the Nurse. Nurses' Medical Practice Problems. Part I. *Amer. J. Nurs.,* **62:**82, (July) 1962.
13. Lesnik, Milton J.: The Board of Nurse Examiners and the Nurse Practice Act. *Amer. J. Nurs.,* **54:**1485, (Dec.) 1954.

14. _____: Nursing Functions and Legal Control. *Amer. J. Nurs.,* **53:**1210, (Oct.) 1953.

15. Meakins, J. C.: Nursing Must Be Defined. *Amer. J. Nurs.,* **48:**622, (Oct.) 1948.

16. Simmons, Leo W., and Henderson, Virginia: *Nursing Research: A Survey and Assessment.* Appleton-Century-Crofts, New York, 1964, p. 461.

17. Goodrich, Annie W.: *The Social and Ethical Significance of Nursing.* The Macmillan Company, New York, 1932, p. 401.

18. Barnes, Elizabeth: *People in Hospital.* Macmillan and Company, Ltd., London, 1961, p. 155. New York, St. Martin's Press.

19. de Hartog, Jan: *The Hospital.* Atheneum, New York, 1964, p. 337.

20. Brown, Esther Lucile: *Newer Dimensions of Patient Care. Part I. The Use of the Hospital for Therapeutic Purposes.* Russell Sage Foundation, New York, 1961, p. 159.

21. _____: *Newer Dimensions of Patient Care. Part II. Improving Staff Motivation and Competence in the General Hospital.* Russell Sage Foundation, New York, 1962, p. 194.

22. _____: *Newer Dimensions of Patient Care. Part III. Patients as People.* Russell Sage Foundation, New York, 1964, p. 163.

23. Jones, Maxwell: *A Therapeutic Community. A New Treatment Method in Psychiatry.* Basic Books, New York, 1956, p. 186.

24. Greenblatt, Milton: *From Custodial to Therapeutic Patient Care.* Russell Sage Foundation, New York, 1955, p. 497.

25. Weiskotten, H. G.: The Present and Future Status of the Hospital Phase of Medical Education. *J. Med. Ed.,* **38:**737, (Sept.) 1963.

26. National League of Nursing Education and National Organization for Public Health Nursing, Joint Committee on Integration of the Social and Health Aspects of Nursing in the Basic Curriculum: *Bibliography on Social and Health Aspects of Nursing in the Basic Curriculum.* The Committee, New York, 1950, p. 14.

27. World Health Organization: *Training the Physician for Family Practice.* Technical Report Series No. 257, The Organization, Geneva, 1963, p. 39.

28. Snoke, P. S., and Weinerman, E. R.: *An Annotated Bibliography on Comprehensive Care Programs in University Medical Centers.* In preparation. Yale University School of Medicine, New Haven, Conn.

29. Schwartz, Doris, *et al.:* The Nurse, Social Worker and Medical Student in a Comprehensive Care Program. *Amer. J. Nurs.,* **58:**39, (Jan.) 1958.

30. _____: *Interim Report on a Study of Nursing Needs of Chronically Ill Ambulatory Patients, over the Age of 60, in a General Medical Clinic.* The Cornell-New York Hospital Medical Center, New York. Research Memorandum No. 10, Series B, (May) 1960, p. 10.

31. Crew, F. A. E.: Nursing as a National Service. The Second Revolution. *Nurs. Times,* **51:**483, (6 May) 1955.

32. Spain, David M.: *The Complications of Modern Medical Practices: A Treatise on Iatrogenic Diseases.* Grune & Stratton, New York, 1963, p. 342.

33. Severdlik, Samuel S., *et al.*: Fifty Years of Progress in Physical Medicine and Rehabilitation in New York State. *New York J. Med.*, **51**:90, (Jan.) 1951.

34. Buchwald, Edith (in collaboration with Howard A. Rusk, George G. Deaver, and Donald A. Covelt): *Physical Medicine for Daily Living*. McGraw-Hill Book Co., New York, 1952, p. 183.

35. Williams, Mary Edna: The Patient Profile. *Nurs. Res.*, **9**:122, (Summer) 1960.

36. National League of Nursing Education. Special Committee on Postgraduate Clinical Courses (Elizabeth K. Porter, Chairman): *Courses in Clinical Nursing for Graduate Nurses. Basic Assumptions and Guiding Principles. Basic Courses. Advanced Courses*. The League, New York, 1945, p. 12.

37. National League of Nursing Education: *A Curriculum Guide for Schools of Nursing*. The League, New York, 1937, p. 689.

38. Tudor, Gwen E.: A Sociopsychiatric Nursing Approach to Intervention in a Problem of Mutual Withdrawal on a Mental Hospital Ward. *Psychiatry,* **15**:193, (May) 1952.

39. Orlando, Ida Jean: *The Dynamic Nurse-Patient Relationship: Function, Process and Principles*. G. P. Putnam's Sons, New York, 1961, p. 91.

40. Yale University School of Nursing: *Self-Evaluating Report of Yale University School of Nursing*. The School, New Haven, 1964, various paging.

41. Wiedenbach, Ernestine: *Clinical Nursing: A Helping Art*. Springer Publishing Co., New York, 1964, p. 118.

42. Dumas, Rhetaugh, *et al.*: Validating a Theory of Nursing Practice. *Amer. J. Nurs.,* **63**:52, (Aug.) 1963.

43. Abdellah, Faye: Methods of Identifying Covert Aspects of Nursing. *Nurs. Res.,* **60**:4, (June) 1957.

44. Hathaway, John S., and Fitzgerald, Helene: A New Dimension to the Nurse's Role. *Nurs. Outlook,* **10**:535, (Aug.) 1962.

45. Henderson, Virginia: *Basic Principles of Nursing Care*. International Council of Nurses, London, 1961, p. 42.

46. Nursing. *Nurs. Times,* **49**:1049, (17 Oct.) 1953.

47. Houston, William R.: *The Art of Treatment*. The Macmillan Co., New York, 1936, p. 744.

48. Saunders, Cecily: Should the Patient Know? *Nurs. Times,* **55**:954, (16 Oct.) 1959.

49. _____: Control of Pain in Terminal Cancer. *Nurs. Times,* **5**:1031, (23 Oct.) 1959.

50. _____: Mental Distress in the Dying. *Nurs. Times,* **55**:1067, (30 Oct.) 1959.

51. Burnett, Florence, *et al.*: Learning the Mental Hygiene Approach Through the Chronic Medical Patient. *Publ. Hlth. Nurs.,* **43**:319, (June) 1951.

52. Harmer, Bertha, and Henderson, Virginia: *Textbook of the Principles and Practice of Nursing,* 5th ed. The Macmillan Co., New York, 1955, p. 1,250.

53. Bochnak, Mary A., et al.: *The Effect of Nursing Activity on the Relief of Pain.* American Nurses Association, New York, 1962 (Monograph No. 6).

54. Rhymes, Julina P.: Nursing to Relieve Distress by Meeting Patients' Needs. *Minnesota Nurs. Accent,* **35**:55, (June) 1963.

55. Yankauer, Ruth Gillen, and Levine, Eugene: The Floor Manager Position—Does It Help the Nursing Unit? *Nurs. Res.,* **3**:4, (June) 1954.

56. Smith, Dorothy M.: Myth and Method in Nursing Practice. *Amer. J. Nurs.,* **64**:68, (Feb.) 1964.

57. ———: A Real Laboratory for Learning. *Nurs. Outlook,* **11**:274, (Apr.) 1963.

58. Turk, Herman, and Ingles, Thelma: *Clinic Nursing. Explorations in Role Innovation.* F. A. Davis, Philadelphia, 1963, p. 192.

59. Flores, Florence: Role of the Graduate Nurse Today. *New England J. Med.,* **267**:487, (6 Sept.) 1962.

60. Weiner, Florence R.: Professional Consequences of the Nurse's Occupational Status. *Amer. J. Nurs.,* **51**:614, (Oct.) 1951.

61. Kreuter, Frances Reiter: What Is Good Nursing Care? *Nurs. Outlook,* **5**:302, (May) 1957.

62. Kroeger, Louis J., *et al.: Nursing Practice in California Hospitals.* California State Nurse's Association, San Francisco, 1953, p. 401.

63. Roth, Julius A.: Ritual and Magic in the Control of Contagion. *Amer. Sociol. Rev.,* **22**:310, (June) 1957.

64. Hillway, Tyrus: *Introduction to Research.* Houghton-Mifflin, Boston, 1956, p. 284.

65. Vreeland, Ellwynne M.: Nursing Research Programs of the Public Health Service. Highlights and Trends. *Nurs. Res.,* **13**:148, (Spring) 1964.

66. Simmons, Leo W., and Henderson, Virginia: *op. cit.,* 16.

67. Bayne-Jones, Stanhope: The Role of the Nurse in Medical Progress. *Amer. J. Nurs.,* **50**:601, (Oct.) 1950.

68. U.S. Surgeon General's Consultant Group on Nursing: *Toward Quality in Nursing. Report of Surgeon General's Consultant Group.* U.S. Government Printing Office, Washington, 1963, p. 73.

69. Jackson, Margaret: Where Should the Nurse Be Trained? 2. In Long-stay Hospitals. *Nurs. Times,* **51**:560, (20 May) 1955.

70. Fox, David J.: A Proposed Model for Identifying Research Areas in Nursing. *Nurs. Res.,* **13**:29, (Winter) 1964.

71. Lasagna, Louis: Statistics, Sophistication, Sophistry and Sacred Cows. *Clin. Res. Proc.,* **3**:185, (Nov.) 1955.

72. Wald, Florence S., and Leonard, Robert C.: Towards the Development of Nursing Practice Theory. *Nurs. Res.,* **13**:309, (Fall) 1964.

73. Brown, Myrtle Irene: Research in the Development of Nursing Theory. *Nurs. Res.,* **13**:109, (Spring) 1964.

74. Kelly, Katherine J., and Hammond, Kenneth R.: An Approach to the Study of Clinical Inference in Nursing. *Nurs. Res.,* **13**:314, (Fall) 1964.

75. Macgregor, Frances C.: Research Potential of Collegiate Nursing Students. Developing a Research Attitude and Creative Imagination. A Preliminary Report. *Nurs. Res.,* **13**:259, (Summer) 1964.

76. Van Doren, Mark: *Liberal Education.* Henry Holt, New York, 1943, p. 186.

77. Joint Committee on Educational Facilities for Nursing of the National League for Nursing and Public Health Service: *Nursing Education Facilities: Programing Considerations and Architectural Guide. Report of Joint Committee on Educational Facilities for Nursing of the National League for Nursing and Public Health Service.* U.S. Government Printing Office, Washington, 1964, p. 88 (USPHS Pub. No. 1180-F-1b).

78. Houston, William R.: *op. cit.,* p. 47.

79. Abdellah, Faye G., et al.: *Patient-Centered Approaches to Nursing.* The Macmillan Co., New York, 1961, p. 205.

80. ANA in Review: ANF Conducts Pilot Study of Nursing Periodical Index. *Amer. J. Nurs.,* **12**:8, (Summer) 1964.

81. Research Reporter. American Nurses Foundation to Conduct Pilot Project on Nursing Index. *Nurs. Res.,* **13**:249, (Summer) 1964.

82. American Nurses Association: *Using and Improving the Keys to Knowledge.* The Association, New York, 1964, various paging.

83. Henderson, Virginia, *et al.: Nursing Studies Index,* Vol. IV, 1957–1959. J. B. Lippincott Co., Philadelphia, 1963, p. 281.

84. Griffin, Gerald, *et al.:* Clinical Nursing Instruction and Closed Circuit TV. *Nurs. Res.,* **13**:196, (Summer) 1964.

85. Lewis, Philip: *Educational Television Guidebook.* McGraw-Hill Book Co., New York, 1961, p. 238.

86. Merrill, I. R.: Closed-Circuit Television in Health Sciences Education. *J. Med. Ed.,* **38**:329, (Apr.) 1963.

87. Westley, Bruce H., and Hornback, May: An Experimental Study of the Use of Television in Teaching Basic Nursing Skills. *Nurs. Res.,* **13**:205, (Summer) 1964.

88. Wilcox, Jane: Closed-Circuit Television: A Tool for Nursing Research. *Nurs. Res.,* **13**:210, (Summer) 1964.

89. Craytor, Josephine K., and Lysaught, Jerome P.: Programmed Instruction in Nursing Education—A Trial Use. *Nurs. Res.,* **13**:323, (Fall) 1964.

90. Hector, Winifred E.: Programmed Learning. A New Teaching Method. *Inter. Nurs. Rev.,* **11**:16, (July–Aug.) 1964.

91. Seedor, Marie M.: Can Nursing Be Taught with Teaching Machines? *Amer. J. Nurs.,* **63**:117, (May) 1963.

92. Nutting, Adelaide M.: *A Sound Economic Basis for Schools of Nursing.* G. P. Putnam's Sons, New York, 1926, p. 372.

93. Goodrich, Annie W.: *op. cit.,* 17.

94. Welch, William H.: Address to the Graduating Class of the Johns Hopkins Hospital School of Nursing, Baltimore, 1916.

95. Beard, Richard Olding: The University Education of the Nurse. In *Fifti-eth Annual Report of the American Society of Superintendents of Training Schools for Nurses, Including Report of the Second Meeting of the American Federation of Nurses.* 1909, p. 111.
96. Lyons, E. P.: The Concern of the Medical School in Nursing Education. In pp. 159–165 of *Thirty-Ninth Annual Report of the National League of Nursing Education.* National League for Nursing, New York, 1933.
97. Robson, H. N.: The Need for a Revolution in the Nursing Profession. *Austral. Nurses J.,* **52:**152, (July) 1954.
98. Lindell, John: Nursing as a Profession. *Austral. Nurses J.,* **52:**2, (Jan.) 1954.
99. Crew, F. A. E.: *op. cit.,* p. 31.
100. Sand, René: The Nurse—Sentinel of Health. *Austral. Nurses J.,* **52:**80, (Apr.) 1954.
101. MacDermot, H. E.: Nursing in Osler's Student Days. *Canad. Nurse,* **46:**222, (Mar.) 1950.
102. Avery, L. M.: Recognition of Professional Status. *Austral. Nurses J.,* **49:**120, (Aug.) 1951.
103. Dennison, Claire: Maintaining the Quality of Service in the Emergency. Nursing Service and Nursing Care Are by No Means Synonymous Terms. *Amer. J. Nurs.,* **42:**774, (July) 1942.